*Nature is an incomparable guide
if you know how to follow her.*

Dr. Carl Jung

First published by
Fame Bright Publishing 2012

Copyright © Robert Morrison

Dr. Robert Morrison asserts the moral right to be identified as the author of this work.

All rights reserved.
No part of this publications may be reproduced, stored in a retrieval system, or transmitted, in any form or by any means, electronic, mechanical, photocopying, recording or otherwise, without the prior permission of the publisher.

ISBN 978-1-4675-1339-5

Graphic project
Laura Finelli

Illustrations
Sarah Opkanum

Photographers
Bruno Ruggiero
Giancarlo Campagnola

Introduction

In an age when health care professionals have come to depend heavily on high-tech diagnostic instrumentation to decipher what is wrong with their patients, practitioners of manual muscle testing continue to rely on the body itself to communicate what it needs and doesn't need. While not designed to replace standard diagnostic procedures, manual muscle testing does serve well as an adjunct to one's chosen health care profession. Moreover, the techniques are timeless as well as universal, and they provide the practitioner with the ability to comprehend patient problems in ways that are just not possible with conventional diagnostic exams.

Manual muscle testing is often described as an evaluation of functional neurology because the tests are used to assess the inner workings of the nervous system as opposed to simply gauging the raw power that individual muscles are able to produce. Changes in "strength" observed in manual muscle testing are a reflection of changes in the central integrative state of the anterior horn motor neuron pool of the muscle being tested. The central integrative state is defined as the summation of all excitatory inputs and inhibitory inputs at the neuron. Therefore, the terms "conditionally facilitated" and "conditionally inhibited" more aptly describe what is commonly referred to as "strong" and "weak" muscles respectively. Seen from this perspective, manual muscle testing is essentially a tool for dialoguing with higher nerve centers: muscles become interpreters that translate information from the body to the examiner.

Historical background

The first published records of diagnostic use of manual muscle testing were those of Dr. Robert W. Lovett, Professor of Orthopedic Surgery at Harvard Medical School. Dr. Lovett was specifically interested in evaluating spinal nerve damage, and in 1932, he published a grading system of 5 levels of muscle strength against gravity and external pressure. Lovett's methods would be refined in the 1930s and 1940s by physical therapists Kendall, Kendall, and Wadsworth as they used manual muscle testing to quantify motor loss in poliomyelitis patients. Over time, Kendall and Kendall expanded their scope and began to advocate the use of manual muscle testing in postural disorders.

A major breakthrough came in 1964 when Michigan chiropractor Dr. George Goodheart, using the techniques of Kendall and Kendall, observed that muscles would often test "weak," even in the absence of atrophy or other frank neurological signs. Probing further, Goodheart noted that those same "weak" muscles would immediately regain "strength" after massaging the nodular areas along their origins with heavy pressure. These findings prompted further investigation into the diagnostic utility of manual muscle testing, and heralded the birth of Applied Kinesiology: a vast system of combined therapies that uses manual muscle testing as one of its primary modes of diagnosis.

Manual muscle testing today

To the dismay of many serious practitioners of manual muscle testing today, "kinesiologist" has become an umbrella term for anyone, level of training notwithstanding, who employs some form of manual muscle testing for any number of purported reasons. It should be clarified, however, that *kinesiology* is, by definition, the scientific study of human movement, not to be confused with "Applied Kinesiology," a complex system of diagnostic and therapeutic protocols. The latter is tightly regulated by the International College of Applied Kinesiology (I.C.A.K.), a body of health care professionals whose major purpose is to provide a forum for practitioners around the world, and to promote research and education.

The triad of health to which Applied Kinesiologists refer is symbolized as an equilateral triangle representing the three interdependent aspects of human health and disease: structure, chemistry, and emotions. Most health care professionals today are oriented around just one of the three sides. Whatever the case may be, manual muscle testing offers an infinite number of practical applications that adaptable to all branches of the healing arts. For example, chiropractors, osteopaths, and physical therapists with the major focus on body structure, utilize manual muscle testing to diagnose and correct neuro-musculo-skeletal disorders such as radiculopathies, muscle imbalances, osseous subluxations, cranial faults, etc. Dentists and orthodontists, also concerned with structure, use manual muscle testing to detect and prevent pathology within the stomatognathic system, and also to implement and modify orthodontic apparatus. The chemical side of the triangle, has long been dominated by medical doctors prescribing pharmaceuticals, but also encompasses non-allopathic professionals such as nutritionists, naturopaths, and virtually anyone involved in the administration of "natural" supplements. Here, manual muscle testing becomes particularly useful for determining which substances best suit the needs of the patient for the time in which the tests are performed. The emotional, or mental side of the triangle, primarily the domain of psychologists and psychiatrists, also includes the multitudes of health care professionals involved in mind-body medicine. A wealth of information regarding a patient's psychological status can be obtained using manual muscle testing to monitor involuntary responses to words, sounds, smells, thoughts, and images.

Finally, there is a fourth category which is not represented within the triad of health, but which nevertheless exists as an inseparable part of human health and disease, namely the realm of electromagnetic energy or what is sometimes referred to as "vibrational" medicine. Professionals in this field would include homeopaths, acupuncturists, and all types of eastern medical practitioners.

Technique

Manual muscle testing is as much an art as it is a science. The experienced practitioner becomes skilled at improvising, and adapting to each individual patient (art), while remaining mindful not to compromise the integrity of the standard methodology (science).

To achieve accurate, reproducible results, the following must remain constant each time a muscle is tested:
- starting point of test
- vector of force

- amount of force
- velocity of force
- the timing in which the force is applied
- the contact points on the patient
- instruction or demonstration to the patient
- the examiner's body position (i.e., posture, position of elbow, arm and forearm, etc.)

The following factors must also be considered when performing manual muscle testing:

- **Keep hands off of the body**: apart from the contacts necessary to perform the test, the patient, examiner, or other third party, must avoid touching the body during testing.

- **Stabilize patient adequately for each test**: use a relatively wide contact with the palm of your hand, as opposed to knife-edge or fingertip contact.

- **Avoid causing pain during the test** (i.e. keep clear of bony contacts).

- **Be alert to patient's attempts to recruit synergist muscles**: isolate each muscle to the maximum in order to prevent patient from compensating with synergists.

- **Avoid contact with electromagnetic devices**: physical contact with cell phones, wristwatches, or other such devices can cause aberrant results.

- **Patient must remain in neutral centered body position with head in midline**.

- **Patient must keep eyes open and in neutral position**.

- **Patient must avoid chewing or clenching teeth**.

- **Patient must keep the mouth free of candy, chewing gum or other substances**.

- **Patient must avoid deep inhalation or exhalation, and refrain from holding their breath, or bearing down during the test**.

- **Patient must avoid grimacing and tensing facial muscles**.

- **Avoid contact with acupuncture points**.

- **Mind contraindications**: i.e., pathology, acute pain, inflammation, etc.

- **Muscle testing is not a contest**: it is not uncommon for either the examiner or patient to feel as though they are competing with each other during muscle testing. When this occurs, it may be necessary to remind the patient (or oneself) that the tests are not a contest, but rather a way of obtaining information from the body.

- **Remain impartial**: be conscious of any preconceived ideas or expectations as to the outcome of any test.

- **Have patient lightly clench their teeth when flexors are tested in the prone position and when extensors are tested in the supine, seated, or standing position**: the tonic labyrinthine reflexes overfacilitate flexors in the prone position and overfacilitate extensors in the supine, seated, and standing positions. By having the patient lightly clench their teeth, the effects of the tonic labyrinthine reflexes are overridden and won't interfere with normal testing.

BOOK FORMAT

Each section includes useful clinical information related to each muscle. Listed below are summaries of each component:

Origin, Insertion, Innervation, Action:
a comprehensive and detailed knowledge of anatomy is critical in order to perform manual muscle testing properly.

Clinical:
this section outlines the clinical significance and classic presentations associated with each muscle.

Chapman reflexes
(a.k.a. Chapman's points or neurolymphatic reflex points):
these are discrete cutaneous tissue texture changes, that correlate to internal dysfunction or pathology.
Dimension and precise location of these points vary from person to person, but they are found consistently at specific sites about the trunk, arms, and thighs. In the 1920^S and 1930^S, osteopath Frank Chapman linked these points to individual viscera and their associated health problems. During the 1960^S, chiropractor Dr. George Goodheart correlated Chapman's reflexes to individual muscles. Where mentioned in this text, the points are assumed to be bilateral, with both anterior and posterior locations (unless specified otherwise). The majority of posterior points are found adjacent to specific vertebral levels and are listed accordingly (i.e., L3, L4, L5, etc.).

Neurovascular point
(a.k.a. Bennett's neurovascular reflexes):
in the 1930^s, chiropractor Terence Bennett described small points about the head and trunk and their relation to the vascular flow of viscera. These points are found both unilaterally and bilaterally, and can be felt with a light fingertip contact as slight pulsations. Bennett's reflexes serve both diagnostic as well as therapeutic function. During the 1960^s, Dr. George Goodheart correlated these points to individual muscles and groups of muscles.

Nutrition:
individual muscles and groups of muscles require specific nutrients.
For example, muscles that support the lower back and pelvis relate to the need for vitamin E while shoulder muscles are generally associated with vitamin C.

Acupuncture meridian association:
electromagnetic energy known as "qi" flows through the body inside 12 bilateral meridians and through the governing and conception vessels found along the midline. In 1966, Dr. George Goodheart integrated these "acupuncture meridian connectors" into Applied Kinesiology after discovering their affiliation with the muscle-organ/gland relations.

Common subluxations:
the term "subluxation" in this book refers to malpositioned or misaligned vertebrae, innominate bones, and sacrum. Subluxations tend to occur at spinal nerve level of "weak" muscles.

Meric TS line:
these refer to two separate systems based on the interaction between soma and viscera. The Meric system, developed by chiropractor B.J. Palmer, links vertebral levels to specific organs and glands. The TS line, first described by chiropractor M.L. Rees, refers to points along Temporo-sphenoidal line that become tender and nodular when there is dysfunction of a corresponding organ or gland. In 1976, Dr. George Goodheart incorporated the TS line

into Applied Kinesiology, after discovering that the points also relate to individual muscles and groups of muscles. The TS line points are found on either side of the cranium and they coincide with the ipsilateral muscles. Diagnostic potential is enhanced when the two systems (Meric system and TS line points) are combined.

Associated point:
there are fourteen associated points, one for each of the twelve meridians and the conception and governing vessels. These points are found adjacent to the spine along the bladder meridian. When active, a vertebral subluxation will usually be present at the corresponding segmental level.
Associated points serve both diagnostic as well as therapeutic function.

Visceral association:
each individual muscle has an associated organ or gland.

Posture:
postural analysis is one of the quickest and most reliable methods for understanding muscle imbalances. Unless stated otherwise, the postural deviations described in this text refer to those which occur when the muscle in question is neurologically inhibited (weak).

Common errors:
familiarity with the common errors will prevent misdiagnoses and subsequent misguided therapy. With experience, the practitioner becomes proficient at recognizing those positions that patients assume while attempting to recruit synergist muscles. Having this knowledge will often enable the examiner to predict the outcome of a test before it is executed.

ACKNOWLEDGEMENTS

I'd like to express gratitude to following people who helped make this book possible: graphic artist Laura Finelli, photographers Bruno Ruggiero and Giancarlo Campagnola, illustrator Sarah Opkanum, models Gianfranco Santoruvo and Francesca Provetti, and to my family for their contributions in proofreading and editing.

Dr. Robert Morrison

CONTENTS

Abdominals	13
Adductors	19
Biceps Brachii	23
Brachioradialis	26
Coracobrachialis	28
Deltoid anterior division	30
Deltoid middle division	32
Deltoid posterior division	34
Extensor Carpi Radialis	36
Extensor Carpi Ulnaris	37
Extensor Digitorum Longus	38
Extensor Hallucis Longus and Brevis	40
Flexor Carpi Radialis	42
Flexor Carpi Ulnaris	43
Flexor Digitorum Longus	44
Flexor Hallucis Longus	45
Gastrocnemeus	47
Gluteus Maximus	51
Gluteus Medius and Minimus	54
Gracilis	57
Hamstrings	60
Iliacus	64
Iliopsoas	66
Infraspinatus	70
Latissimus Dorsi	72
Levator Scapula	75
Medial Neck Flexors	77
Neck Extensors	80
Opponens Digiti Minimi	84
Opponens Pollicis	85
Pectoralis Major Clavicular	87
Pectoralis Major Sternum	90
Pectoralis Minor	93
Peroneus Brevis	95
Peroneus Longus	97
Peroneus Tertius	99
Piriformis	101
Popliteus	104
Posterior Tibialis	106
Pronator Quadratus	108
Pronator Teres	110
Quadratus Lumborum	112
Quadriceps	114
Rhomboids	120
Sacrospinalis	122
Sartorius	125
Serratus Anterior	128
Soleus	131
Sternocleidomastoid	133
Subscapularis	137
Supinator	140
Supraspinatus	142
Tensor Fascia Lata	144
Teres Major	147
Teres Minor	150
Tibialis Anterior	152
Trapezius Lower Division	154
Trapezius Middle Division	157
Trapezius Upper Division	160
Triceps Brachii	163

ABDOMINALS

The abdominal muscles are made up of the Rectus Abdominis, Transverse Abdominis, Abdominal External Oblique, and Abdominal Internal Obliques.

Transverse Abdominis
Origin: internal surfaces of 7th to 12th costal cartilages; thoracolumbar fascia; anterior three quarters of internal edge of iliac crest; lateral third of inguinal ligament.
Insertion: linea alba with aponeurosis of internal oblique, pubic crest, and pecten pubis via conjoint tendon.
Action: compresses and supports abdominal viscera in standing position; assists in forced expiration.

Rectus Abdominis
Origin: pubic symphysis and pubic crest.
Insertion: xyphoid process and 5th to 7th costal cartilages.
Action: flexes trunk; supports abdominal viscera in standing position; holds rib cage and pubis together; gives anterior support to the lumbar spine; with the aid of gluteus maximus, keeps pelvis from going into anterior tilt.

External Oblique Abdominis
Origin: external surfaces of ribs 4 to 12; the 5 superior attachments interdigate with the serratus anterior, and the lower 3 interdigate with latissimus dorsi and their attachments.
Insertion: linea alba; pubic tubercle; anterior half of iliac crest.
Action: compresses and supports abdominal viscera in standing position; gives anterior support to the lumbar spine; flexes vertebral column and draws pubis toward xyphoid process; assists rectus abdominis in obtaining anterior pelvic stability with the gluteus maximus; unilateral action assists in lateral bending, or rotates the vertebral column, bringing the ipsilateral shoulder anteriorly.

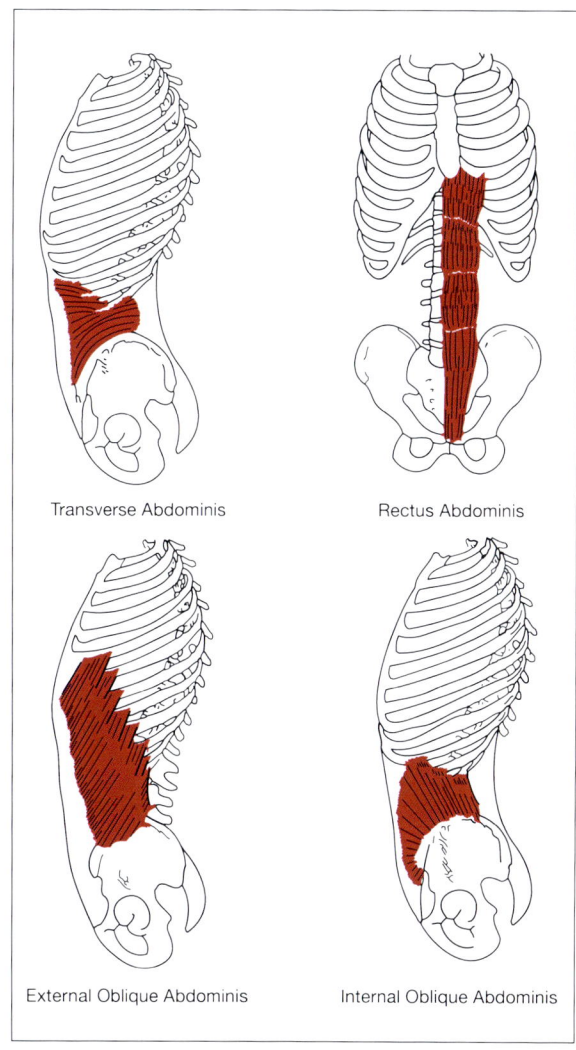

Transverse Abdominis   Rectus Abdominis

External Oblique Abdominis   Internal Oblique Abdominis

Internal Oblique Abdominis
Origin: thoracolumbar fascia; anterior two-thirds of iliac crest; lateral half of inguinal ligament.
Insertion: inferior borders of ribs 10 to 12; linea alba; pubis via the conjoint tendon.
Action: compresses and supports abdominal viscera in standing position; gives anterior support to the lumbar spine; flexes lumbar spine and draws pelvis and thorax together; laterally flexes and rotates vertebral column bringing the contralateral shoulder anteriorly.

ABDOMINALS

CLINICAL*

General Abdominals
- low back pain
- difficulty flexing trunk, touching toes, and sitting up from a lying down position
- narcolepsy
- duodenal "dumping syndrome"
- paroxysms of sneezing
- on rare occasion, found to be weak contralateral to "frozen shoulder"
- weakness is associated with sagittal suture jamming
- hyperlordosis associated with bilateral weakness (bilateral gluteus maximus weakness)
- sway back posture

Rectus Abdominis
- difficulty lifting head off table

Oblique Abdominals
- difficulty turning body (rotating thorax) i.e., skiing, hitting a tennis ball, looking over shoulder in car
- internal obliques - pain in testicle (cremasteric muscle)
- internal obliques - inguinal hernia

Transverse Abdominis
- lateral abdominal wall bulges during sitting

*Courtesy of Drs. Walter Schmitt and Kerry McCord - Quintessential Applications: A(K) Clinical Protocol (QA)

The following applies to all divisions of the abdominal muscles

Innervation
ventral rami of T5-T12 iliohypogastric and ilioinguinal nerves

Chapman's reflexes
Anterior: medial thigh
Posterior: L5/PSIS

Neurovascular point
parietal eminences 2 inches posterior to frontal parietal suture

Nutrition
vitamin E
duodenal substance

Acupuncture meridian association
small intestine

Common subluxations
T5-T12

Meric TS line
T6 and T7

Associated point
S1 and sacroiliac joint (small intestine)

Visceral association
small intestine

ABDOMINALS

POSTURE

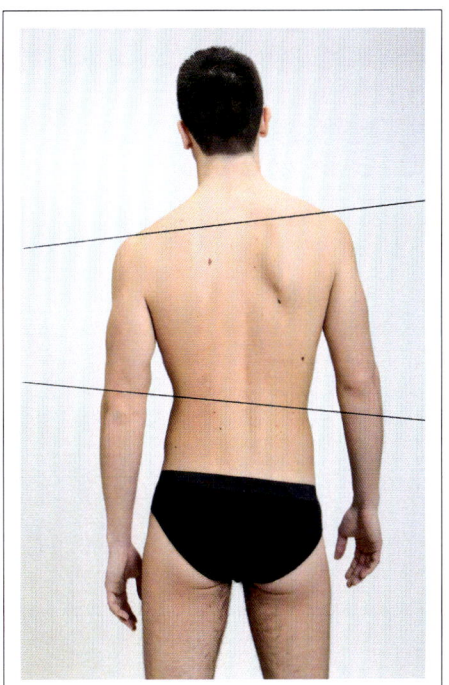

General Abdominals
unilateral weakness: elevated hip and low shoulder on side opposite to weakness.

Transverse Abdominis
lateral abdominal wall bulges and lumbar spine is concave on side of weakness.

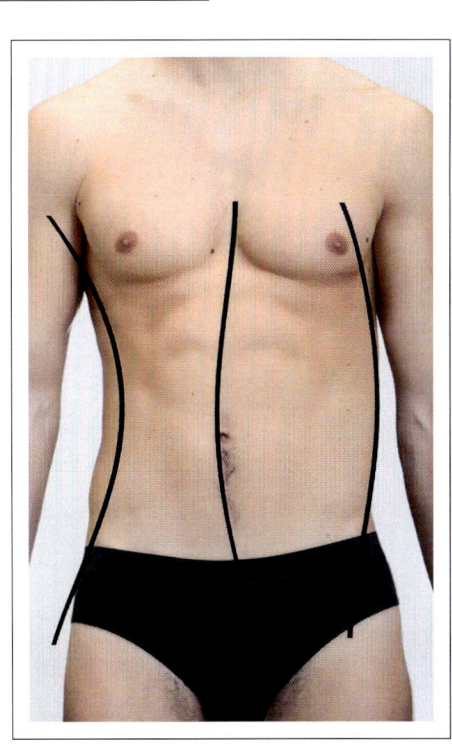

General Abdominals
bilateral weakness: sway back posture or hyperlordosis.

ABDOMINALS

General Abdominals Test

Position
Seated with legs and feet on table.

Test
Patient is seated on table with legs extended along table, hips flexed to approximately 70 degrees, and knees slightly bent.
The spine is kept as straight as possible and the arms are crossed over chest, with closed fists resting over anterior shoulders (to avoid therapy localization).

Examiner stabilizes by placing a hand or forearm over the thighs or over the shins - depending on the relative strength of examiner and patient - while the other hand contacts the posterior surface of the outermost forearm and directs force straight back toward trunk extension.

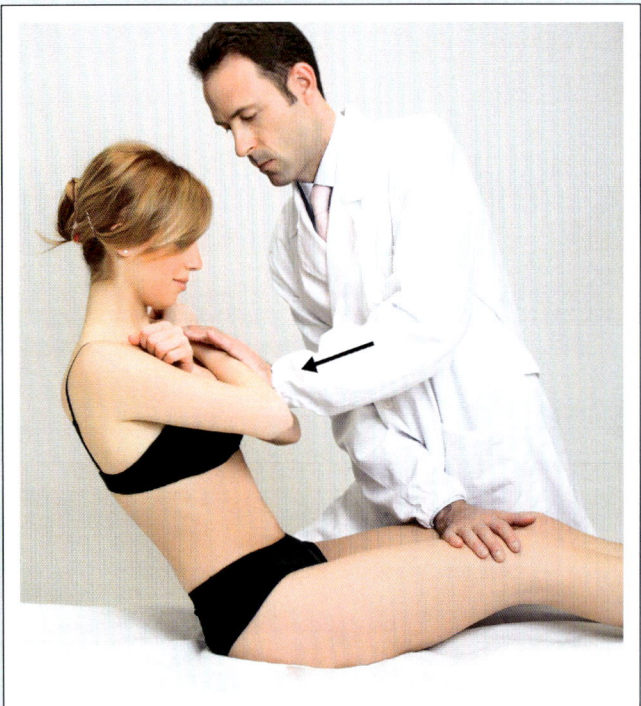
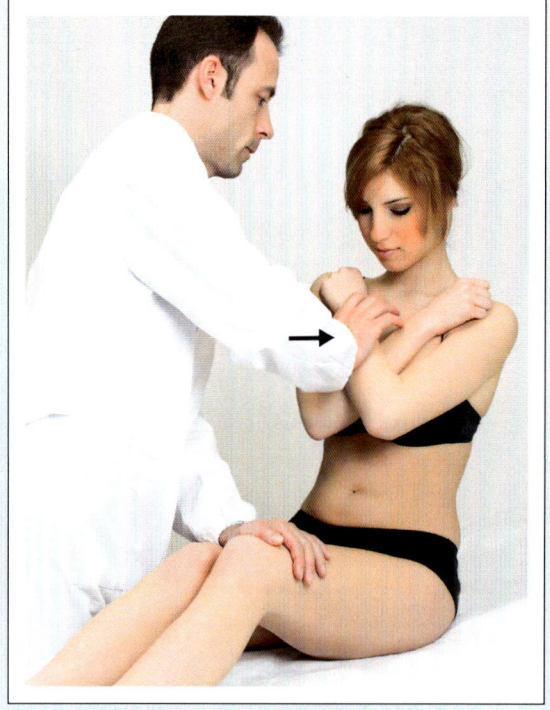

ABDOMINALS

Common errors

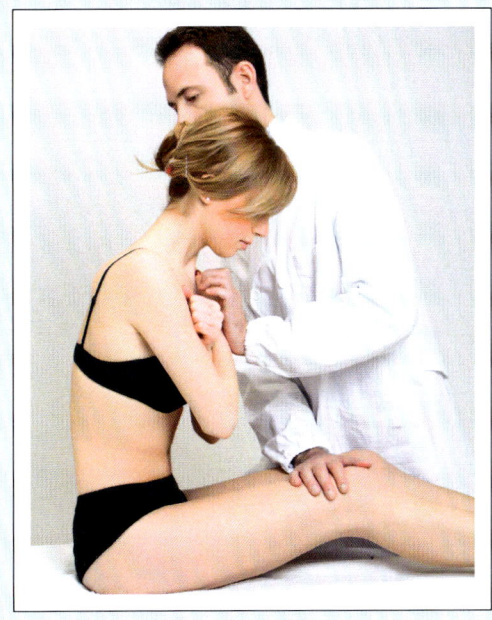
Spine is flexed or starting position is too far forward.

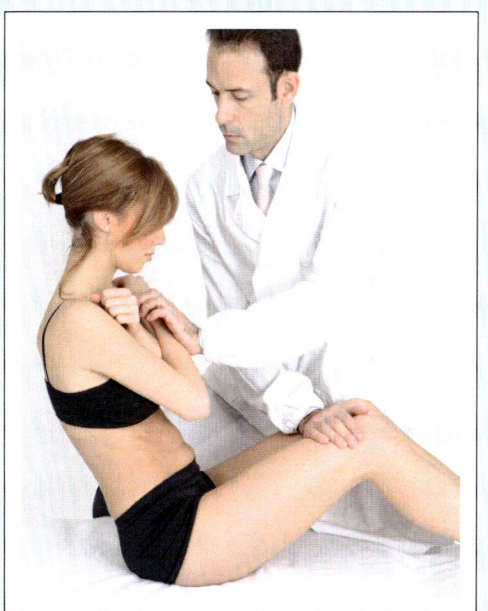
Too much flexion at the hips.

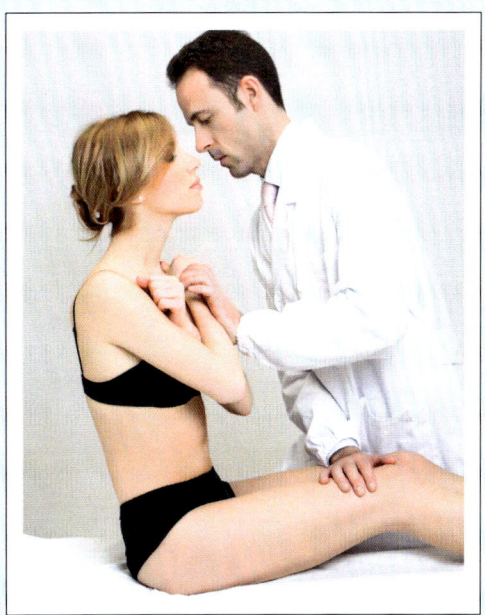
Substitution with neck flexors.

ABDOMINALS

Rectus Abdominis Test

Position
Seated with legs and feet on table.

Test
Patient is seated with legs extended along table, hips flexed to approximately 70 degrees, and knees slightly bent. The spine is kept as straight as possible and the arms are crossed over chest, closed fists resting over anterior shoulders (to avoid therapy localization).
Examiner stabilizes with one hand over the ipsilateral, distal thigh, while the other hand is placed on the posterior surface of the outermost forearm to direct force straight back toward trunk extension.

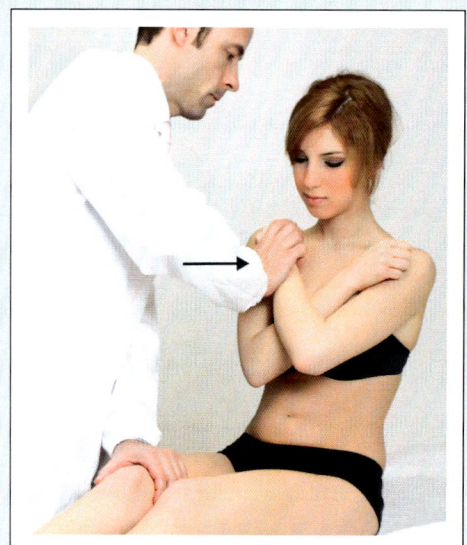

Oblique Abdominals Test

Position
Seated with legs and feet on table.

Test
Patient is seated with legs extended along table, hips flexed to approximately 70 degrees, and knees slightly bent. With the arms crossed, fists resting over anterior shoulders (to avoid therapy localization), patient maximally rotates the spine to one side. Examiner stands on the opposite side to which the patient has rotated and stabilizes with a hand or forearm on the thighs or shins, while the other hand contacts the lateral surface of the ipsilateral humerus to direct force posteriorly in line with the shoulders. In this way the ipsilateral external obliques and the contralateral internal obliques are tested simultaneously.

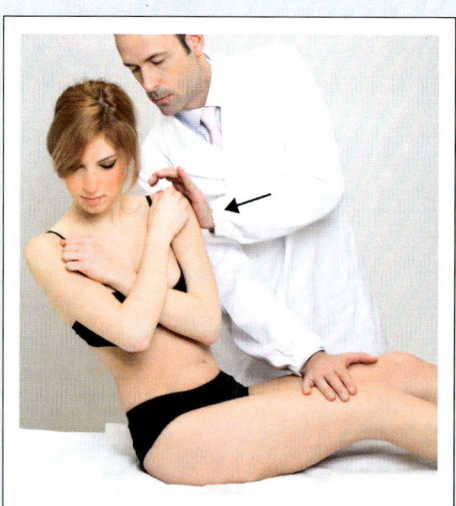

In the above example, the left external abdominal obliques and the right internal abdominal obliques are being tested simultaneously.

ADDUCTORS

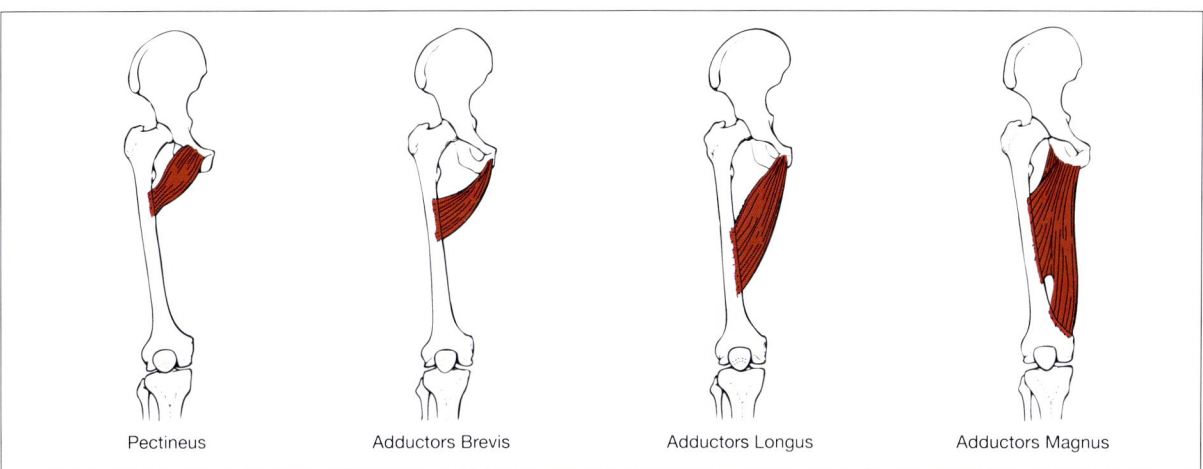

Pectineus | Adductors Brevis | Adductors Longus | Adductors Magnus

The adductor muscles are divided into Pectineus, Adductor Brevis, Adductor Longus, and Adductor Magnus.

Pectineus
Origin: superior surface of pubis.
Insertion: pectineal line of femur from lesser trochanter to linea aspera.
Action: adduction, flexion, and internal rotation of femur.

Adductor Brevis
Origin: body and inferior ramus of pubis.
Insertion: pectineal line and proximal part of linea aspera of femur.
Action: adducts femur with some assistance in flexion.

Adductor Longus
Origin: body of pubis inferior to pubic crest.
Insertion: middle third of linea aspera of femur.
Action: adducts femur with some assistance in flexion.

Adductor Magnus
Origin posterior fibers: ischial tuberosity.
Origin anterior fibers: ramus of ischium and pubis.
Insertion: a line that runs from the greater trochanter along linea aspera, medial supracondylar line, and ending at the adductor tubercle of the medial condyle of the femur.
Action: adducts femur; fibers arising from ischium and ramus of ischium assist in extension of femur while fibers arising from ramus of pubis aid in flexion of femur.

CLINICAL*

- difficulty crossing legs
- medial thigh pain (origin-insertion injuries of adductor magnus)
- difficulty with hip flexion
- lower groin pain
- tight in positive FABER Patrick's sign (weak on opposite side)
- elbow problems (common Chapman's reflex)
- thumb problems (common Chapman's reflex)
- category 2 ilium (LiLL)

*Courtesy of Drs. Walter Schmitt and Kerry McCord Quintessential Applications: A(K) Clinical Protocol (QA)

ADDUCTORS

Innervation
Pectineus: obturator and femoral (L2-L4)
Adductor Brevis: obturator (L2-L4)
Adductor Longus: obturator (L2-L4)
Adductor Magnus: obturator and sciatic (L2-S1)

Chapman's reflexes
Anterior: anterior chest wall behind areola (not in breast tissue)
Posterior: below inferior angle of scapula

Neurovascular point
on lambdoidal suture between lambdoid and asterion

Nutrition
vitamin E;
male or female organ gland substance

Acupuncture meridian association
circulation sex (pericardium)

Common subluxations
(L2-sacrum)

Meric TS line
L5

Associated point
T4, T5 (circulation sex)

Visceral association
reproductive organs and glands

POSTURE

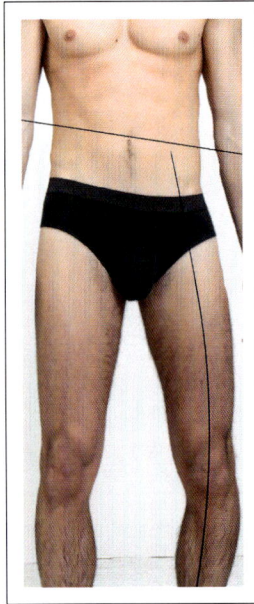

Unilateral weakness: genu varus; contralateral pelvic elevation.

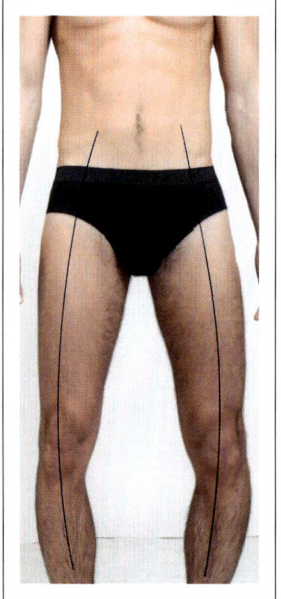

Bilateral weakness: genu varus (bowed legs).

ADDUCTORS

Test 1

Position
Side-lying.

Test
Patient lies on side with entire body straight and the leg to be tested in contact with the table. Examiner stands behind patient and abducts the patient's non-tested leg by pulling up toward the ceiling. This is done in order to get the leg out of the way of the test. With both knees kept in full extension, patient adducts the femur on the side to be tested. Examiner then contacts the medial, distal portion of the same femur, or leg, and directs pressure toward abduction (straight down toward the table).

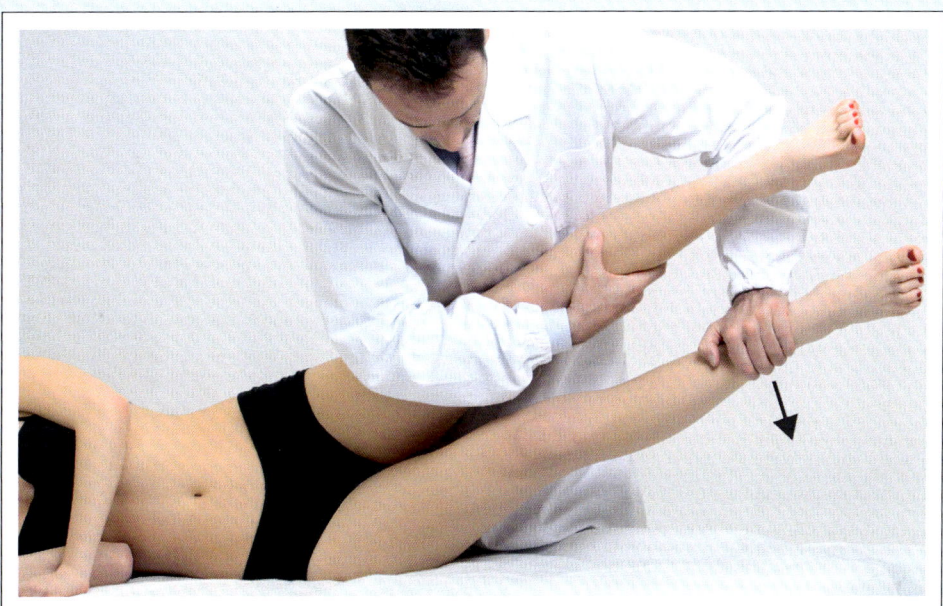

Common error

Poor stabilization in side-lying test allows patient's trunk and pelvis to rotate.

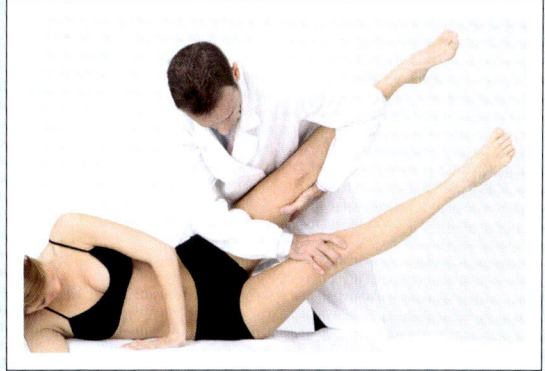

ADDUCTORS

Test 2

Position
Supine.

Test
Keeping both knees locked in extension, supine patient externally rotates the femur on the side being tested to about 20 or 30 degrees.
Examiner stands at the foot of the table and uses one hand to stabilize the lower leg of the non-tested side.

The other hand then contacts the medial, distal leg on the side being tested and pulls away from the midline, using the leg as a lever to impart pressure toward abduction and slight extension of the femur.

N.B. The degree of femur external rotation and the vector of test pressure can vary slightly depending on which adductor muscle is being tested.

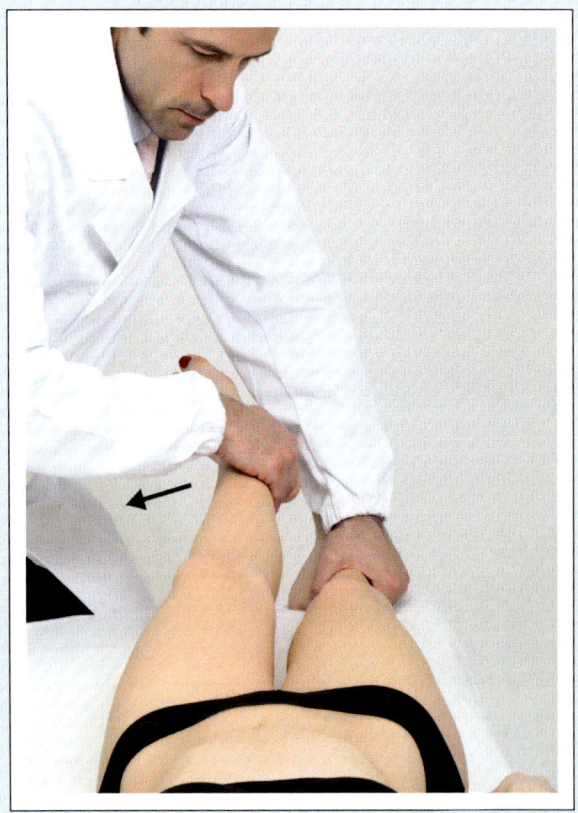

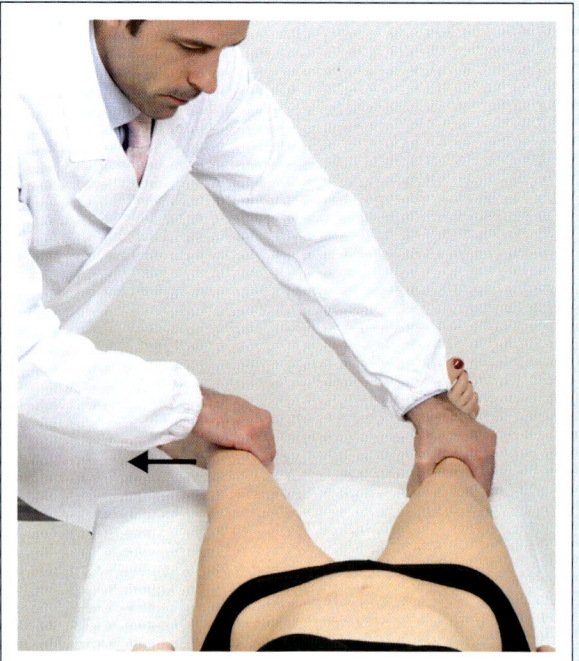

BICEPS BRACHII

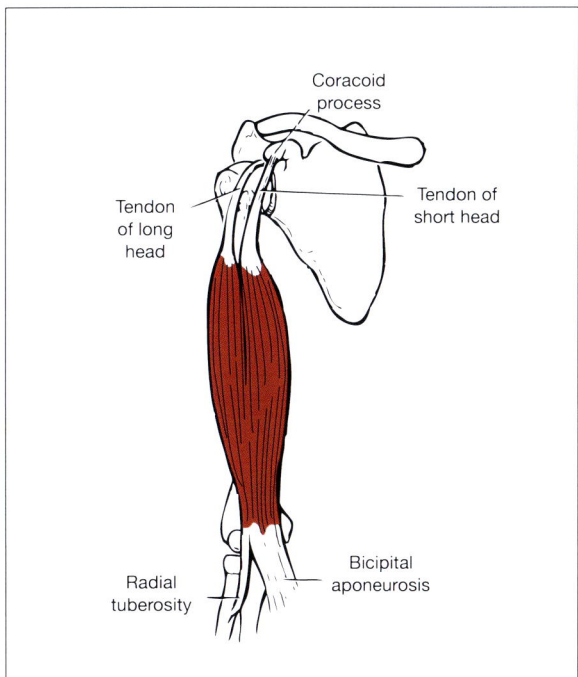

Biceps Brachii

Origin long head: supraglenoid tubercle of scapula.

Origin short head: tip of coracoid process.

Insertion: tuberosity of the radius and fascia of forearm via bicipital aponeurosis.

Action: flexes forearm and humerus and supinates forearm when the motion is resisted.

Chapman's reflexes
Anterior: 4th and 5th intercostal space
Posterior: C2 (T4-T5)

Neurovascular point
frontal bone eminences

Nutrition
betaine hydrochloride; duodenal substance; chlorophyll substance

Acupuncture meridian association
stomach

Common subluxations
C5, C6

Meric TS line
T5

Associated point
T12, L1 (stomach)

Visceral association
stomach

CLINICAL*

- slipped bicipital tendon
- bilateral weakness and/or bilateral shoulder problems induced by hyperinsulinism
- radius subluxations
- difficulty (pain, limited range of motion) on elbow flexion
- difficulty (pain, limited range of motion) on forearm supination especially against resistance
- pain and difficulty using a screwdriver
- long head can rupture at origin (classic "popeye" sign)

*Courtesy of Drs. Walter Schmitt and Kerry McCord
Quintessential Applications: A(K) Clinical Protocol (QA)

BICEPS BRACHII

Test

Position
Seated or supine.

Test
Patient fully supinates forearm and flexes elbow to approximately 45 degrees. Examiner uses one hand to stabilize the posterior, distal humerus, while the other hand contacts the anterior, distal forearm and directs pressure toward extension.

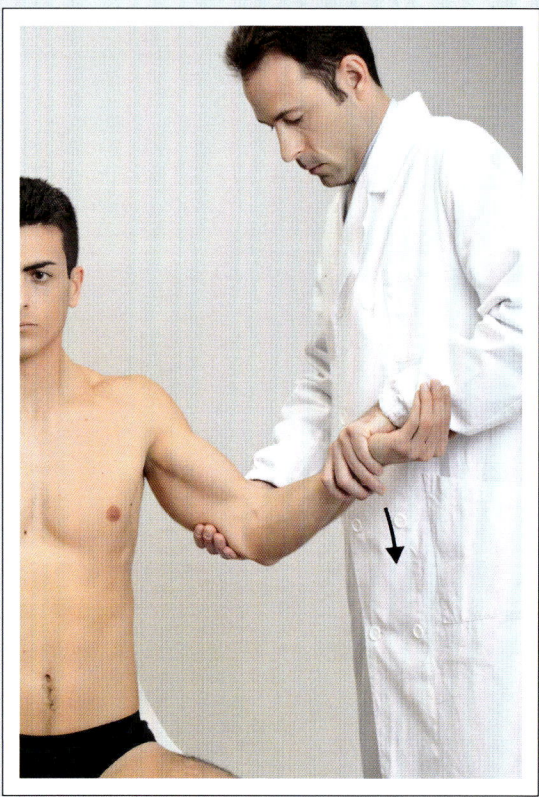

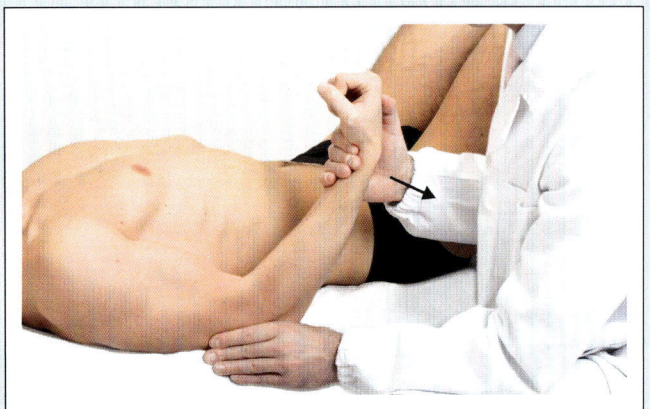

Common error

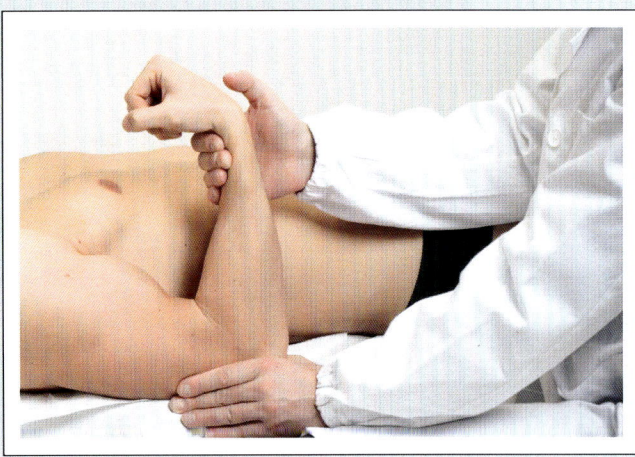

Excess forearm flexion.

BICEPS BRACHII

Biceps Long Head Test

Position
Seated or supine.

Test
Patient locks forearm in full extension and slightly abducts and flexes humerus to about 70-80 degrees.
Examiner uses one hand to stabilize the ipsilateral shoulder, while the other hand contacts the distal, anterior forearm and directs pressure toward extension and slight adduction.

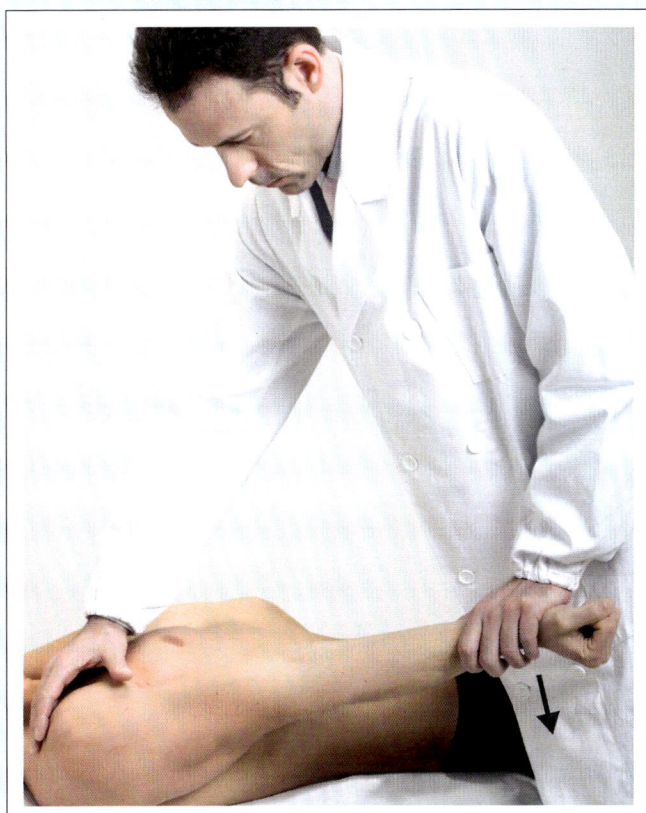
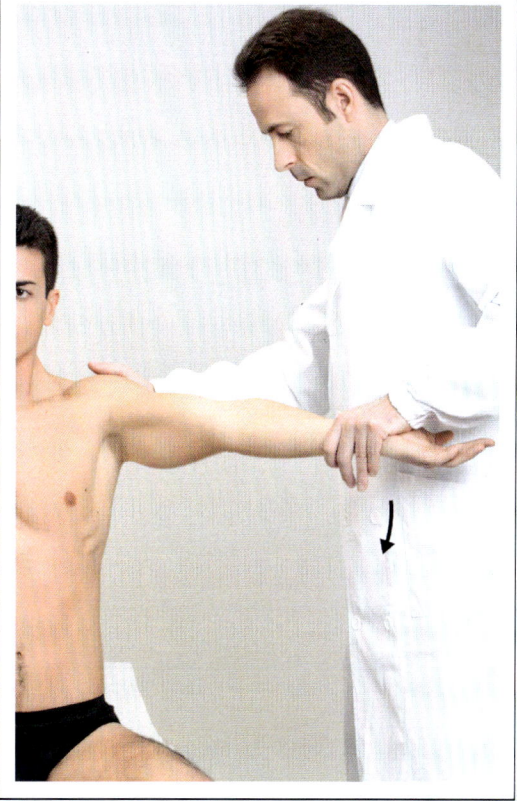

BRACHIORADIALIS

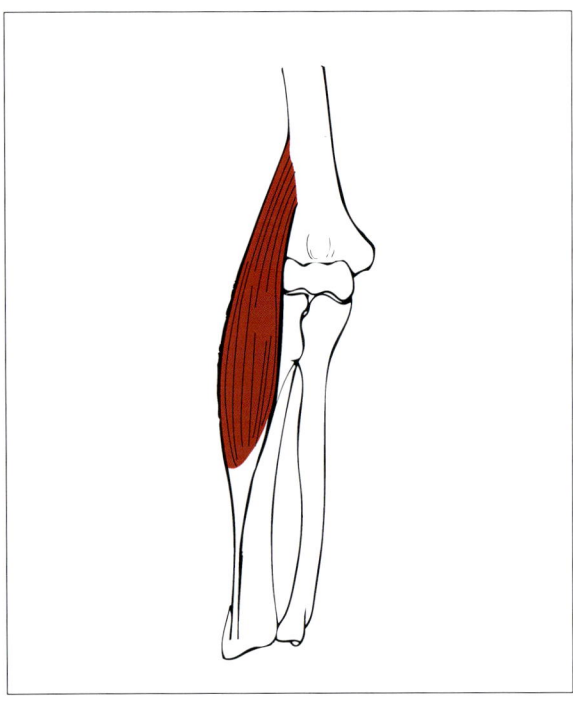

Brachioradialis
Origin: proximal two-thirds of the lateral supracondylar ridge of the humerus and lateral intermuscular septum.

Insertion: lateral surface of the radial styloid process.

Innervation: radial nerve (C5-C6).

Action: flexes semi-pronated forearm; aids in supination in the pronated position and vice versa.

CLINICAL*

- elbow pain (usually at origin)
- pain/fatigue when holding weight with arm in semi-pronated position
- associated with general nervous tension and anxiety

*Courtesy of Drs. Walter Schmitt and Kerry McCord
Quintessential Applications: A(K) Clinical Protocol (QA)

Chapman's reflexes
Anterior: entire pectoralis major muscle
Posterior: over supraspinatus

Acupuncture meridian association
stomach

Associated point
T12, L1 (stomach)

Visceral association
stomach

BRACHIORADIALIS

Test

Position
Seated or supine.

Test
Patient flexes forearm to about 75 degrees keeping it in neutral rotation with thumb pointing cephalad. Examiner stabilizes at the posterior, distal humerus with one hand, while the other hand contacts the lateral surface of the distal forearm and directs pressure toward extension.

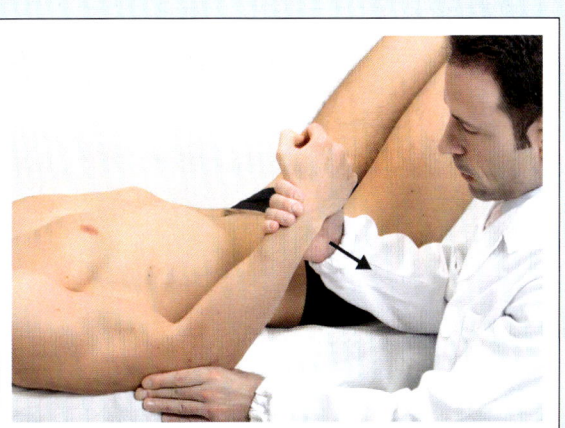

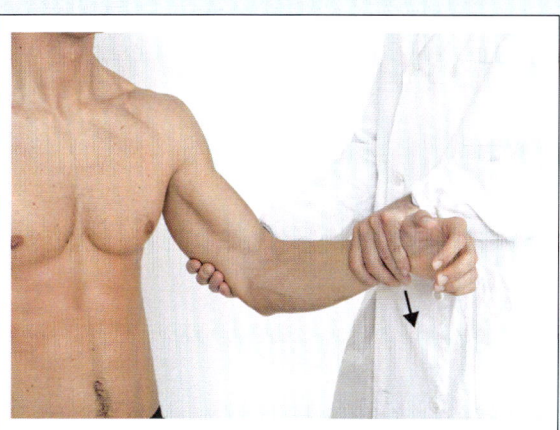

Common errors

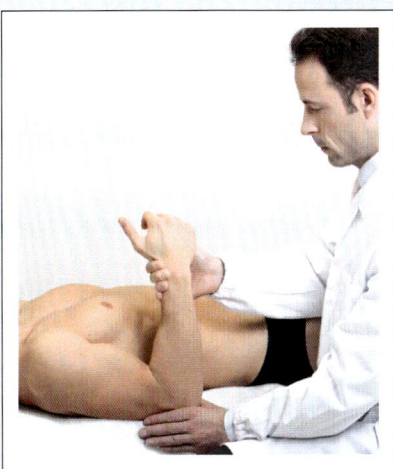

Too much forearm flexion.

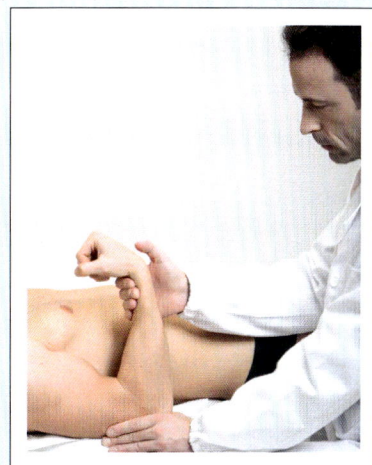

Improper forearm rotation.

CORACOBRACHIALIS

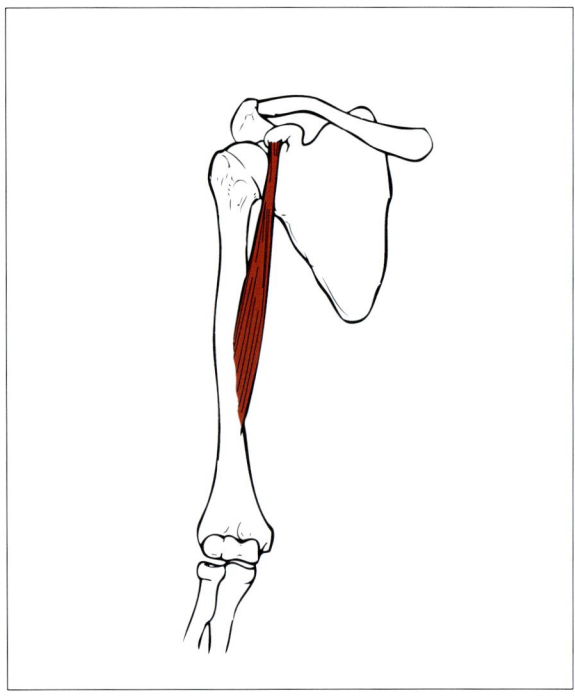

Coracobrachialis
Origin: tip of coracoid process of scapula.

Insertion: middle-third of the medial surface of the humerus.

Innervation: musculocutaneous nerve (C6-C7).

Action: adducts and flexes humerus.

Chapman's reflexes
Anterior: 2nd, 3rd, 4th and 5th intercostal spaces
Posterior: T3, T4, and T5

Neurovascular point
bregma

Nutrition
vitamin C
lung substances

Acupuncture meridian association
lung

Common subluxations
C6 and C7

Meric TS line
T3

Associated point
T3 and T4 (lung)

Visceral association
lungs

CLINICAL*

- difficulty combing hair
- difficulty shaving
- difficulty holding arm up over head
- lung

*Courtesy of Drs. Walter Schmitt and Kerry McCord
Quintessential Applications: A(K) Clinical Protocol (QA)

CORACOBRACHIALIS

Test

Position
Supine or seated.

Test
Patient fully flexes forearm, abducts humerus to about 70 degrees, and flexes humerus to about 70 degrees, adding slight external rotation of the humerus.

Examiner uses one hand to stabilize the posterior, ipsilateral shoulder while the other hand contacts the antero-medial, distal humerus and directs pressure toward extension and slight abduction.

N.B. In testing this muscle, it is useful to remember to first bring the origin and insertion together for the starting position of the test, then to direct test pressure in line with the muscle fibers.

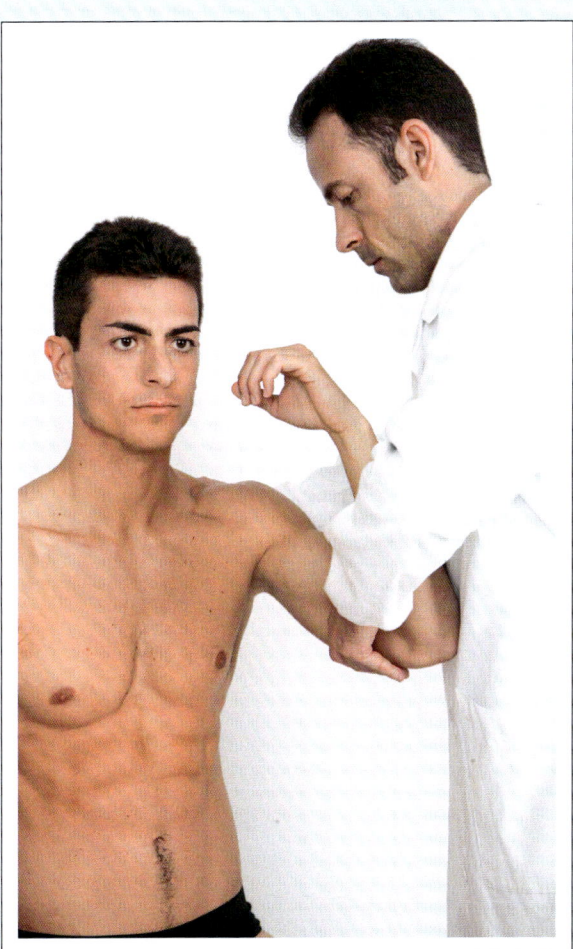

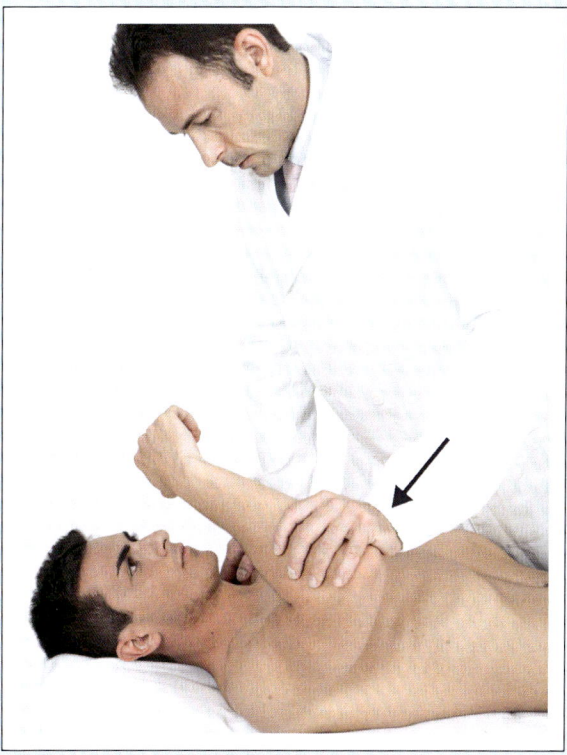

DELTOID ANTERIOR DIVISION

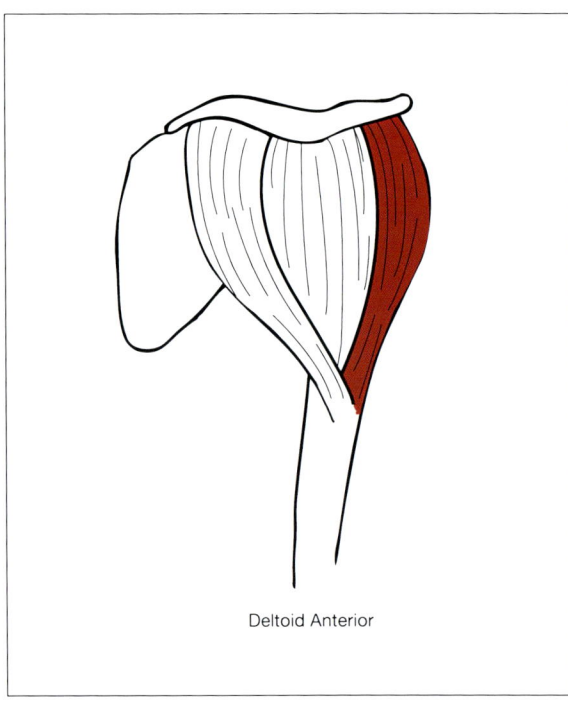

Deltoid Anterior

Deltoid anterior division
Origin: lateral one-third of clavicle on its anterosuperior border.

Insertion: deltoid tubercle of humerus.

Innervation: axillary (C5-C6).

Action: abduction, flexion and internal rotation of humerus.

Chapman's reflexes
Anterior: 2nd, 3rd, 4th and 5th intercostal spaces
Posterior: T3, T4, and T5

Neurovascular point
bregma

Nutrition
vitamin C
lung substances
RNA

Acupuncture meridian association
lung

Common subluxations
C5 and C6

Meric TS line
T3

Associated point
T3 and T4 (lung)

Visceral association
lungs

CLINICAL*

- difficulty with abduction and flexion
- problems throwing
- sometimes associated with gallbladder

*Courtesy of Drs. Walter Schmitt and Kerry McCord Quintessential Applications: A(K) Clinical Protocol (QA)

DELTOID ANTERIOR DIVISION

POSTURE

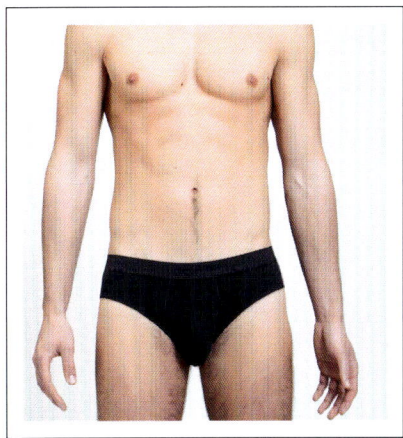

Arm, forearm and hand hang in external rotation. The palm will either face forward or in less extreme cases, the hand will rotate externally from the frontal plane.

Common error

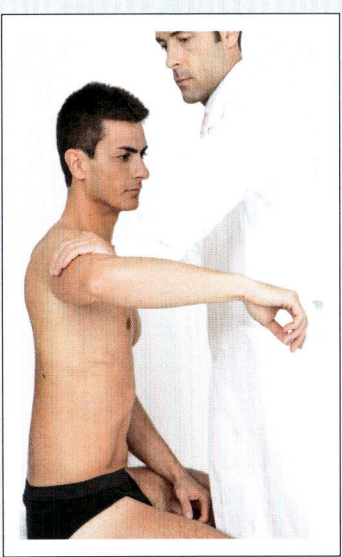

Inadequate arm rotation.

Test

Position
Supine or seated.

Test
Patient abducts humerus to 90 degrees, flexes forearm to 90 degrees, and externally rotates humerus to approximately 45 degrees. Examiner stabilizes opposite shoulder with one hand while the other hand contacts the antero-lateral surface of the distal humerus and directs pressure toward adduction and slight extension.

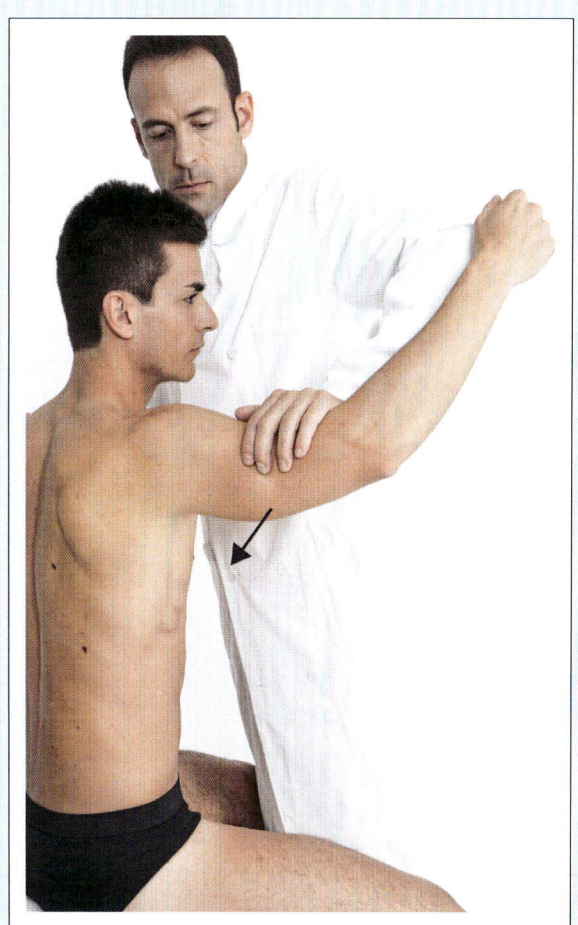

DELTOID MIDDLE DIVISION

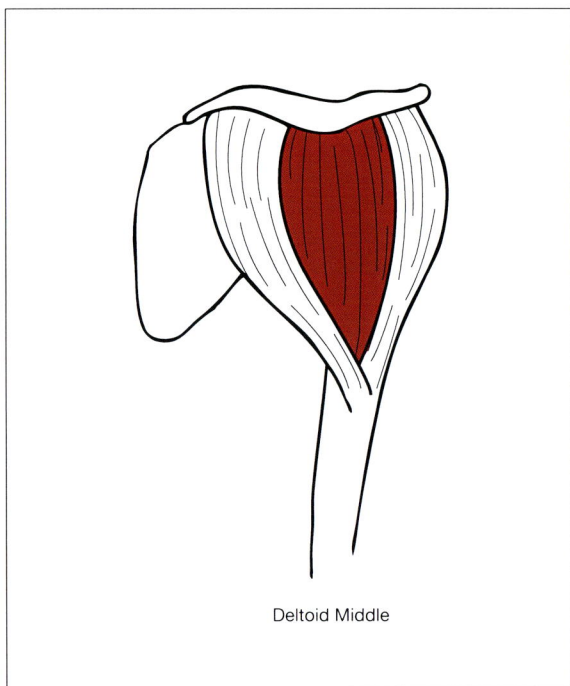

Deltoid Middle

Deltoid middle division
Origin: superior surface of acromion.

Insertion: deltoid tubercle of humerus.

Innervation: axillary (C5-C6).

Action: abduction of humerus.

Chapman's reflexes
Anterior: 2nd, 3rd, 4th and 5th intercostal spaces
Posterior: T3, T4, and T5

Neurovascular point
bregma

Nutrition
vitamin C
lung substances
RNA

Acupuncture meridian association
lung

Common subluxations
C5 and C6

Meric TS line
T3

Associated point
T3 and T4 (lung)

Visceral association
lungs

CLINICAL*

- difficulty with shoulder abduction
- absent lung sounds pneumothorax
- lung conditions
- less likely in asthma
- route of elimination
- nasal sinus congestion
- C7-T2 fixations

*Courtesy of Drs. Walter Schmitt and Kerry McCord
Quintessential Applications: A(K) Clinical Protocol (QA)

DELTOID MIDDLE DIVISION

Test

Position
Supine or seated.

Test
Patient abducts humerus to 90 degrees and flexes arm to 90 degrees. Examiner stabilizes contralateral shoulder with one hand while the other hand contacts the lateral surface of the distal humerus and directs pressure toward adduction.

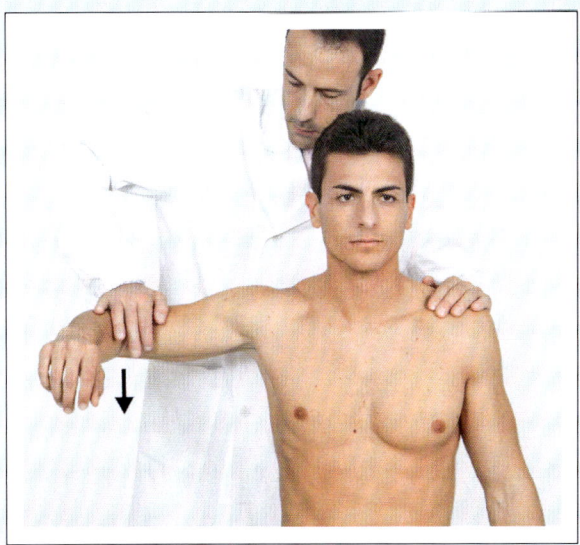

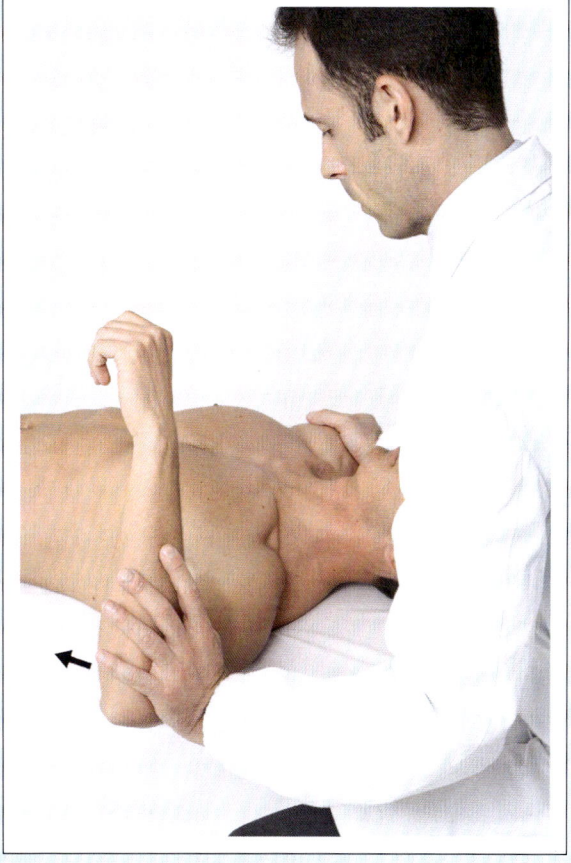

Common error

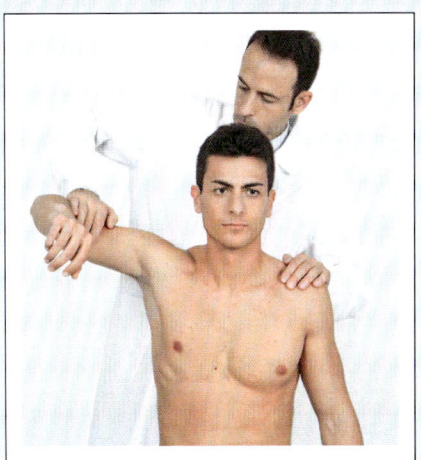

Too much abduction.

DELTOID POSTERIOR DIVISION

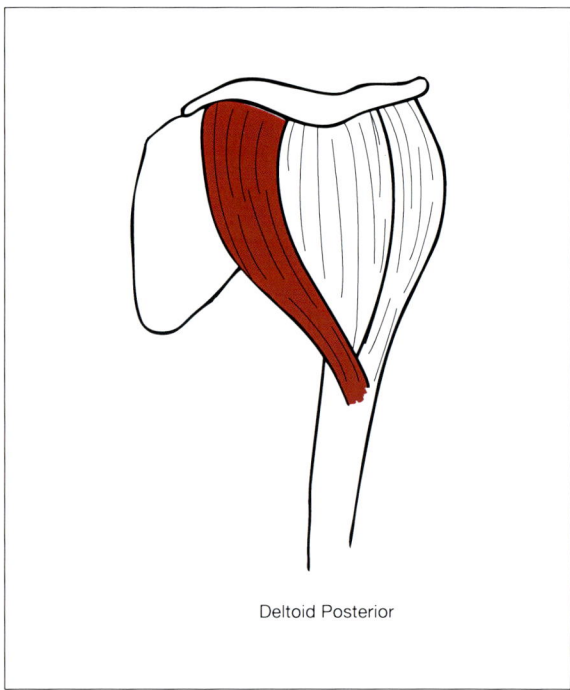

Deltoid Posterior

Deltoid posterior division
Origin: inferior lip of spine of scapula.

Insertion: deltoid tubercle of humerus.

Innervation: axillary (C5-C6).

Action: abduction, slight extension, and external rotation of humerus.

Chapman's reflexes
Anterior: 2nd, 3rd, 4th and 5th intercostal spaces
Posterior: T3, T4, and T5

Neurovascular point
bregma

Nutrition
vitamin C
lung substances
RNA

Acupuncture meridian association
lung

Common subluxations
C5 and C6

Meric TS line
T3

Associated point
T3 and T4 (lung)

Visceral association
lungs

CLINICAL*

- injured with supraspinatus
- difficulty with abduction and reaching backward
- difficulty with adduction from an abducted position

*Courtesy of Drs. Walter Schmitt and Kerry McCord
Quintessential Applications: A(K) Clinical Protocol (QA)

DELTOID POSTERIOR DIVISION

POSTURE

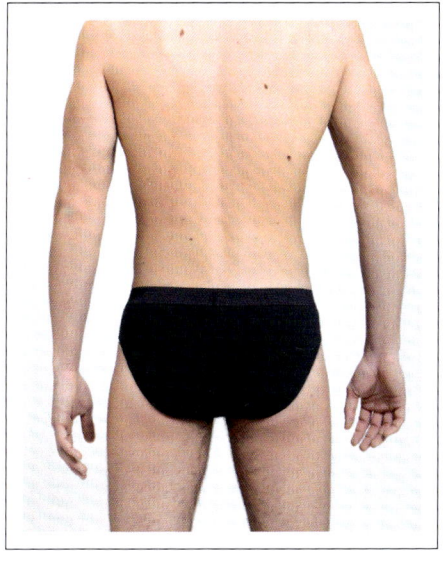

Arm, forearm, and hand hang in internal rotation (palm faces backward).

Test

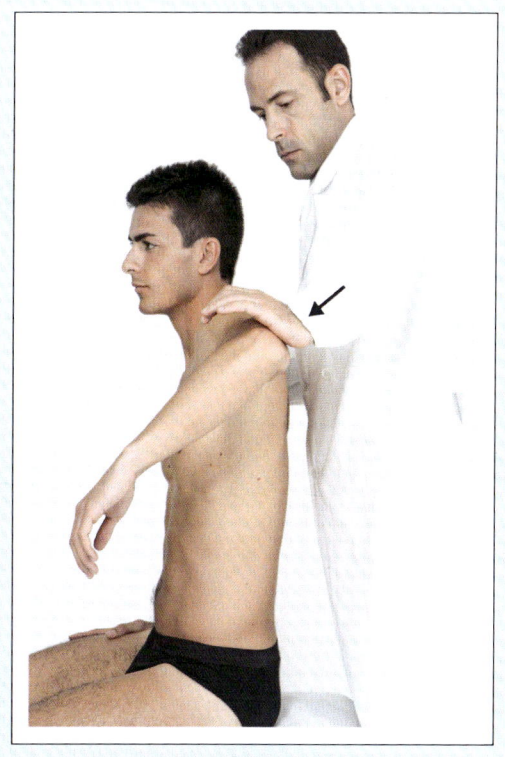

Position
Supine or seated.

Test
Patient abducts humerus to 90 degrees, flexes forearm to 90 degrees, and internally rotates humerus to approximately 45 degrees. Examiner stabilizes opposite shoulder with one hand while the other hand contacts the posterior surface of the distal humerus and directs pressure toward adduction and slight flexion.

EXTENSOR CARPI RADIALIS
LONGUS AND BREVIS

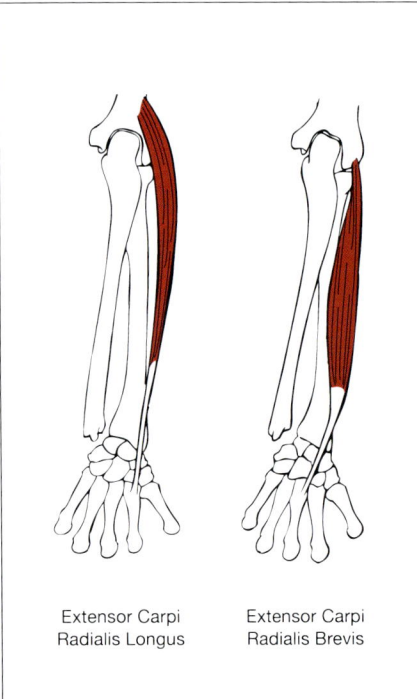

Extensor Carpi Radialis Longus

Extensor Carpi Radialis Brevis

Extensor Carpi Radialis Longus and Brevis
ECR Longus Origin: lateral supracondylar ridge.
Insertion: base of second metacarpal bone.
ECR Brevis Origin: lateral epicondyle of humerus.
Insertion: base of third metacarpal bone.
Innervation (both): radial (C6-C7).
Action (both): extend and radially deviate hand.

CLINICAL*

- elbow problems
- lateral epicondylitis ("tennis elbow")
- pain and limited range of motion on wrist extension
- open ileocecal valve syndrome

*Courtesy of Drs. Walter Schmitt and Kerry McCord
Quintessential Applications: A(K) Clinical Protocol (QA)

Test

Extensor Carpi Radialis Longus and Brevis are tested together.

Test
With teeth lightly clenched, patient flexes the proximal interphalangeal joints and maximally extends the wrist. Examiner contacts the second and third distal metacarpals on the dorsum of the hand and directs pressure toward flexion.

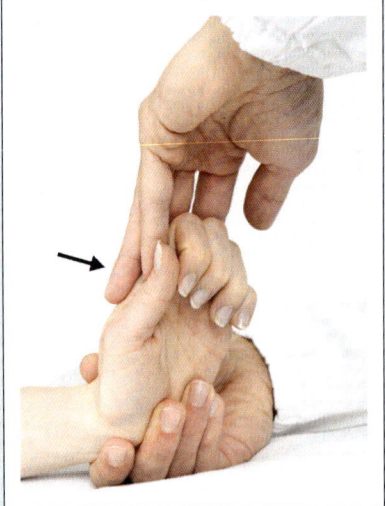
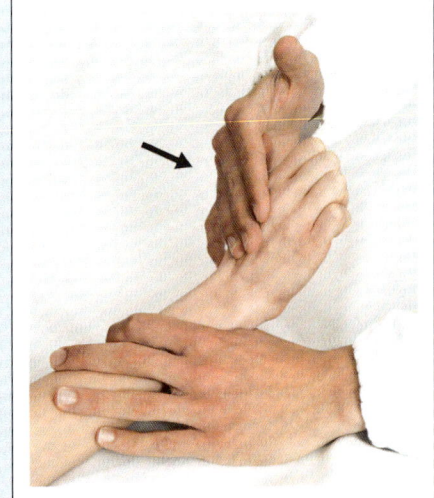

EXTENSOR CARPI ULNARIS

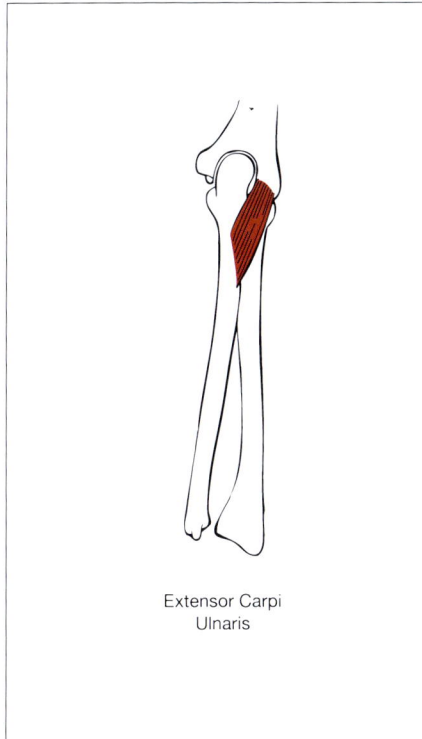

Extensor Carpi Ulnaris

Extensor Carpi Ulnaris
Origin: lateral epicondyle of humerus and posterior border of ulna.
Insertion: base of 5th metacarpal bone.
Innervation: radial (C7-C8).
Action: ulnar deviation and extension of the wrist.

CLINICAL*

- elbow problems
- lateral epicondylitis ("tennis elbow")
- pain and limited range of motion on wrist extension
- open ileocecal valve syndrome

*Courtesy of Drs. Walter Schmitt and Kerry McCord
Quintessential Applications: A(K) Clinical Protocol (QA)

Test

Test
With teeth lightly clenched, patient flexes the proximal interphalangeal joints and maximally extends the wrist. Examiner contacts the the ulnar side of the dorsum of the hand over the fifth metacarpal and directs pressure toward flexion.

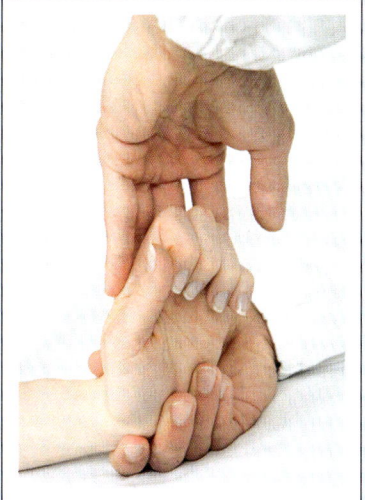
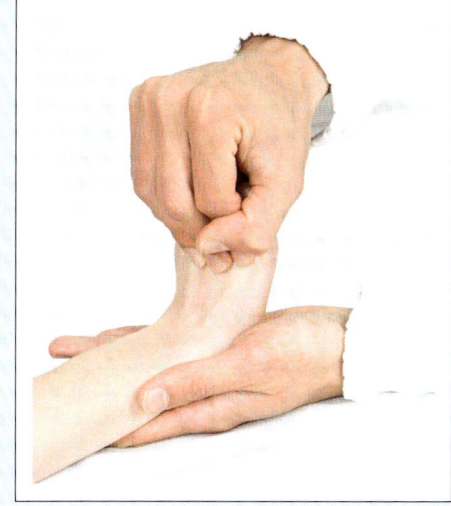

EXTENSOR DIGITORUM LONGUS

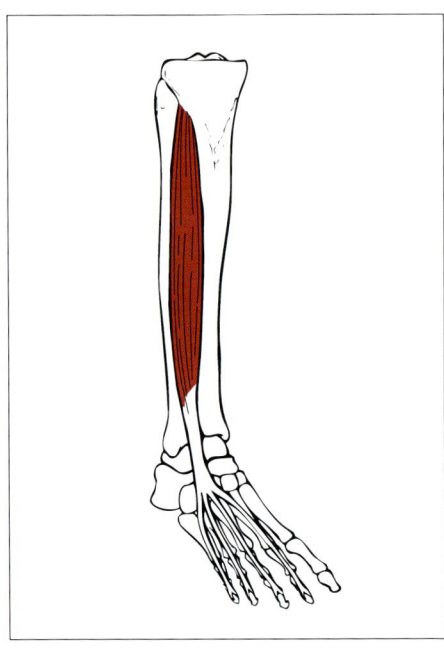

Extensor Digitorum Longus

Origin: lateral tibial condyle; proximal three-fourths of anterior fibula; interosseous membrane; deep fascia; intermuscular septum.

Insertion: medial and lateral sides of toes 2 through 5.

Innervation: peroneal (L4-S1).

Action: extends toes; assists in foot dorsiflexion and eversion.

Test 1

Position
Supine or seated.

Test
Examiner stabilizes foot in slight plantar flexion with one hand while patient lightly clenches teeth, holds the foot in slight plantar flexion and extends toes. Examiner contacts the dorsal surfaces of toes 2 through 5 and directs pressure toward flexion.

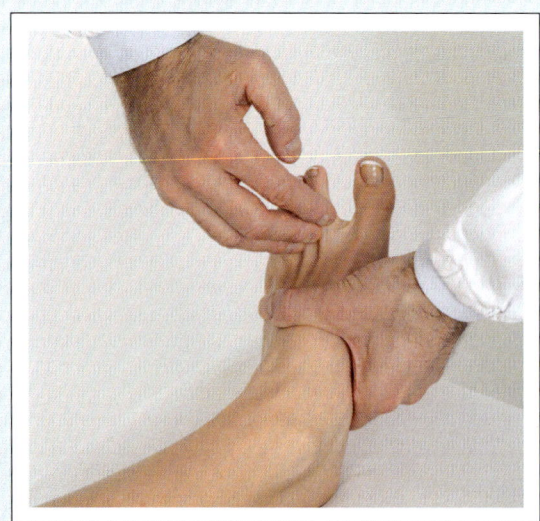

EXTENSOR DIGITORUM LONGUS

Alternate Test 1

Position
Supine or seated.

Test
Patient lightly clenches teeth, holds the foot in slight plantar flexion and extends toes. Examiner stabilizes the big toe with a pincer contact of one hand while the fingers of the other hand contact the dorsal surfaces of toes 2 through 5 to direct pressure toward flexion.

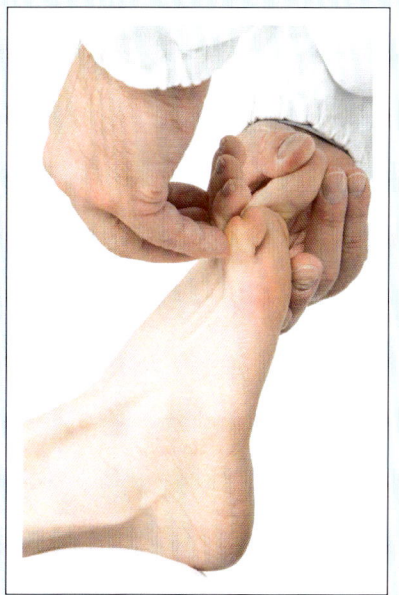

Alternate Test 2

Position
Supine or seated.

Test
Patient lightly clenches teeth and holds the foot in slight plantar flexion.
Examiner stabilizes the big toe by holding it in the web of his thumb and index finger and with the same index finger the proximal phalanges are stablized along the plantar surfaces. The fingers of the other hand are then used to contact the dorsal surfaces of distal phalanges 2 through 5 to direct pressure toward flexion.

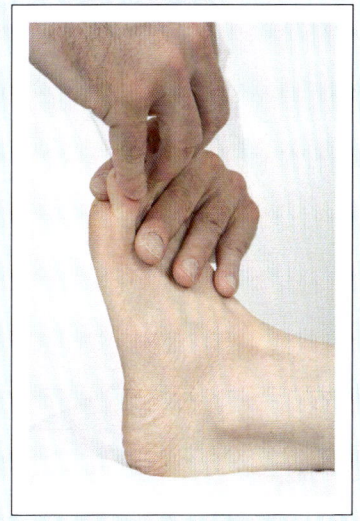
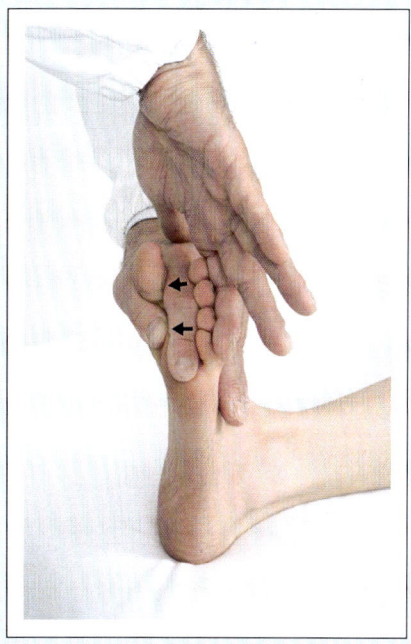

EXTENSOR HALLUCIS
LONGUS AND BREVIS

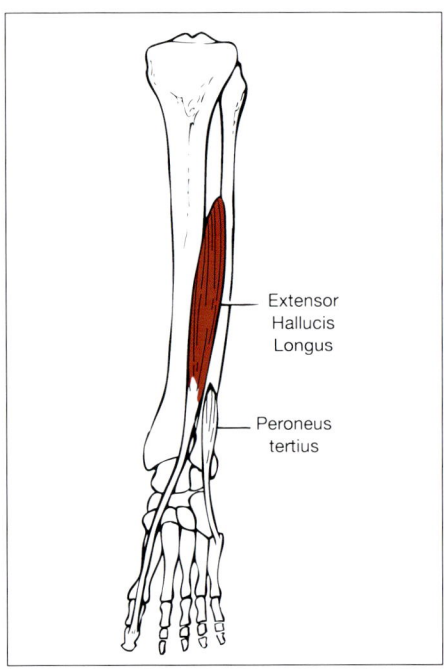

Extensor Hallucis Longus

Origin: middle part of the anterior surface of the fibula and interosseous membrane.

Insertion: dorsal aspect of the base of distal phalanx of great toe.

Innervation: peroneal (L5-S1).

Action: extends great toe and dorsiflexes foot.

Extensor Hallucis Longus Test

Position
Supine.

Test
Patient lightly clenches teeth and holds foot midway between dorsiflexion and plantarflexion. Examiner uses a pincer contact of one hand to stabilize the proximal phalanx of the great toe then in any number of ways, the fingers of either hand contact the dorsal surfaces of toes 2 through 5 in order to prevent extension. Finally, a finger tip contact is made at the dorsal surface of the distal phalanx of the great toe and pressure is directed toward flexion.

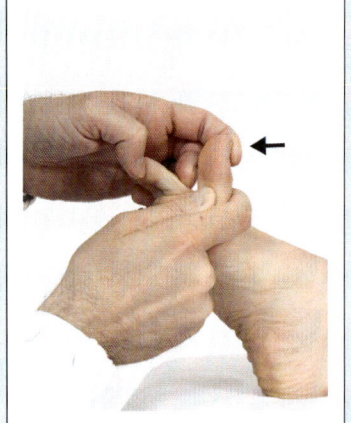
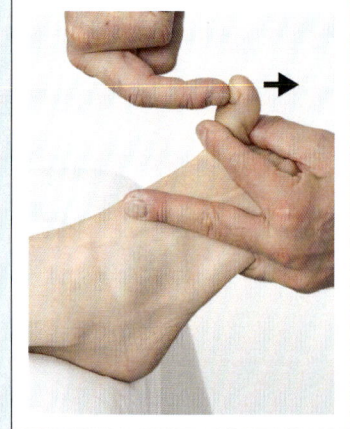

EXTENSOR HALLUCIS LONGUS AND BREVIS

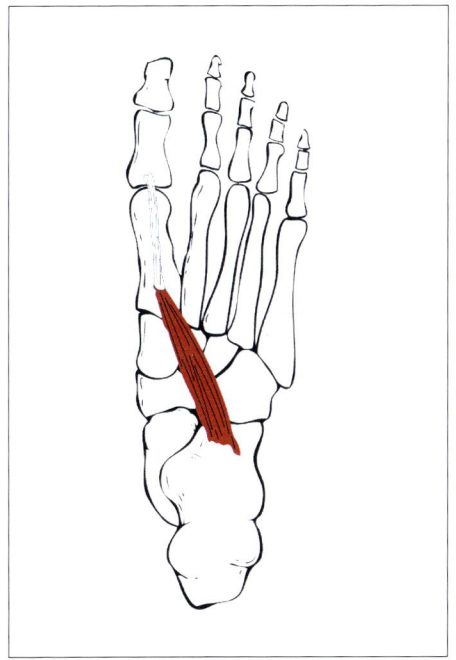

Extensor Hallucis Brevis

Origin: superior lateral surface of anterior calcaneus.

Insertion: proximal phalanx of the great toe.

Innervation: peroneal (L5-S1).

Action: extends great toe at the proximal phalanx.

Test for Extensor Hallucis Longus and Brevis together

Position
Supine.

Test
Patient lightly clenches teeth and holds foot midway between dorsiflexion and plantarflexion.
Examiner uses the fingers of one hand to keep digits 2 through 5 in flexion while the other hand contacts the dorsal surface of the proximal phalanx of the great toe and pressure is directed toward flexion.

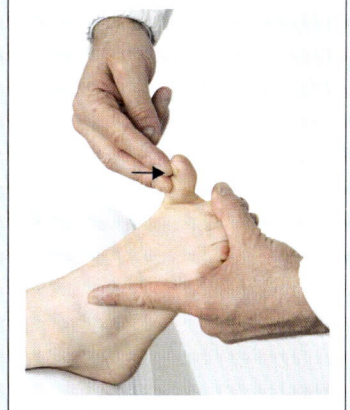
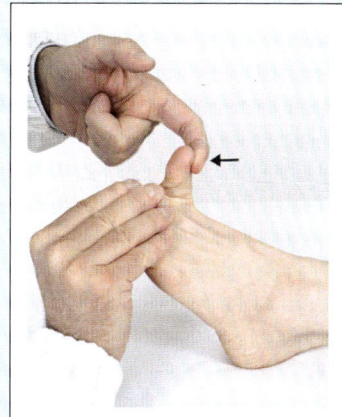

FLEXOR CARPI RADIALIS

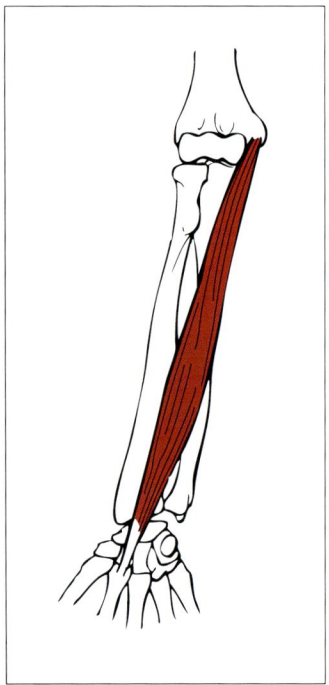

Flexor Carpi Radialis
Origin: medial epicondyle of humerus.
Insertion: base of second metacarpal bone.
Innervation: median (C6-C7).
Action: wrist flexion and slight radial deviation; stabilizes wrist for finger movements.

CLINICAL*

- elbow pain
- medial epicondylitis ("golf elbow")
- wrist pain
- weakness on flexion

*Courtesy of Drs. W. Schmitt and K. McCord
Quintessential Applications:
A(K) Clinical Protocol (QA)

Chapman's reflexes
Anterior: anterior chest wall behind areola (not in breast tissue)
Posterior: below inferior angle of scapula

Test

Holding fingers straight, patient flexes and radially deviates wrist. Examiner contacts thenar eminence and directs pressure toward extension and slight ulnar deviation.

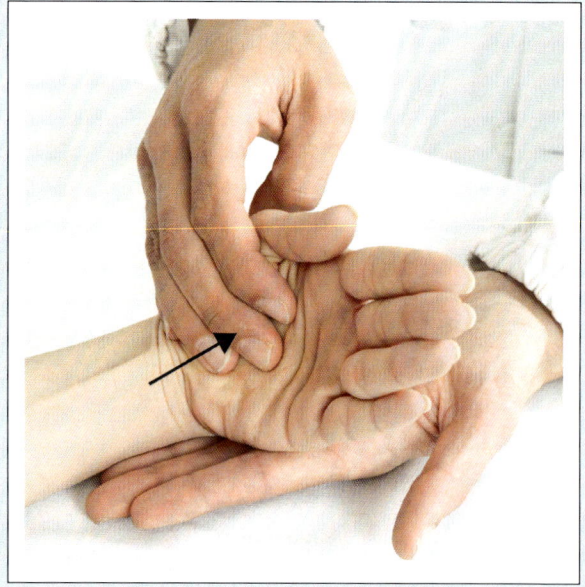

FLEXOR CARPI ULNARIS

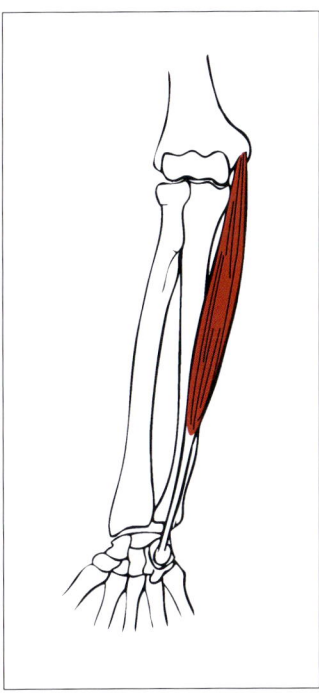

Flexor Carpi Ulnaris
Origin humeral head: medial epicondyle of humerus.
Origin ulnar head: olecranon and posterior border of ulna.
Insertion: pisiform bone.
Innervation: ulnar (C7-C8).
Action: flexes and ulnar deviates wrist.

CLINICAL*

- elbow pain
- medial epicondylitis ("golf elbow")
- wrist pain
- weakness on flexion

*Courtesy of Drs. W. Schmitt and K. McCord
Quintessential Applications:
A(K) Clinical Protocol (QA)

Chapman's reflexes
Anterior: anterior chest wall behind areola (not in breast tissue)
Posterior: below inferior angle of scapula

Test

Holding fingers straight, patient flexes and ulnar deviates wrist. Examiner contacts hypothenar eminence and directs pressure toward extension and slight radial deviation.

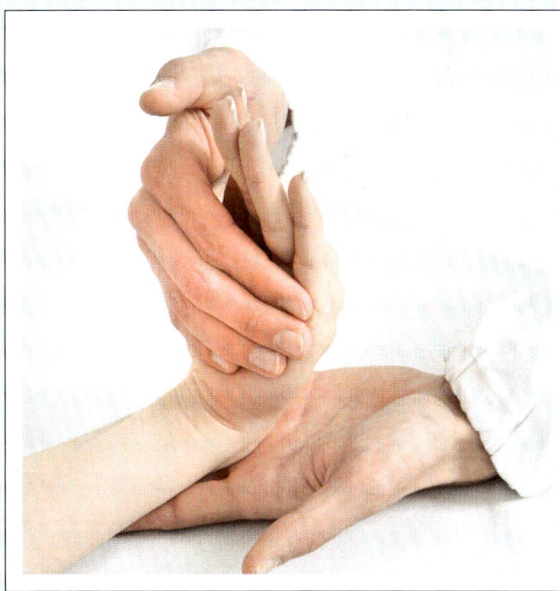

FLEXOR DIGITORUM LONGUS

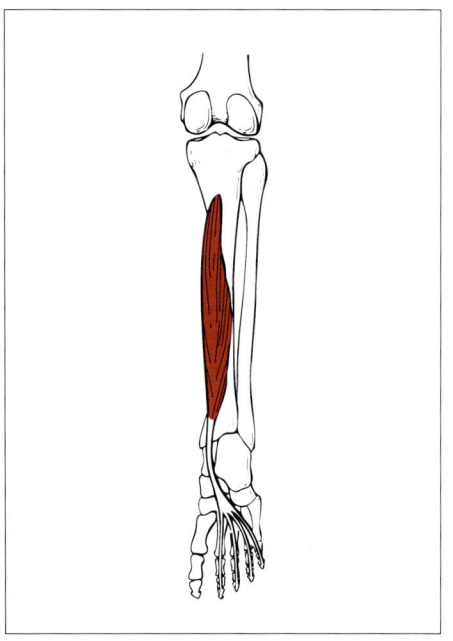

Flexor Digitorum Longus

Origin: medial part of posterior surface of tibia, inferior to soleal line, and by a broad aponeurosis to fibula.

Insertion: plantar surface bases of distal phalanges of lateral four digits.

Innervation: tibial (S2-S3).

Action: flexes lateral four digits and plantarflexes foot; supports longitudinal arch of foot.

Test

Position
Supine.

Test
Patient holds the foot in slight plantarflexion. Examiner stabilizes the great toe in the web of his index and middle fingers positioning the same index finger along the dorsal surfaces of the proximal phalanges 2 through 5 in order to prevent dorsiflexion. Patient flexes toes 2 through 5. Examiner contacts the distal, plantar surfaces of toes 2 through 5 and directs pressure toward extension.

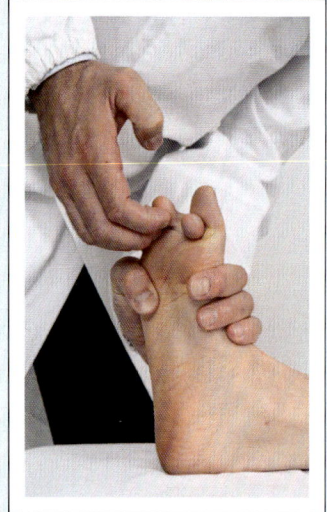
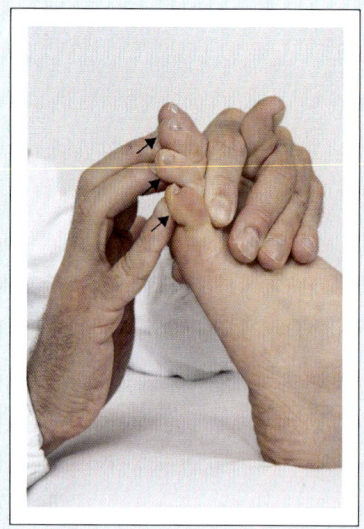

FLEXOR HALLUCIS LONGUS

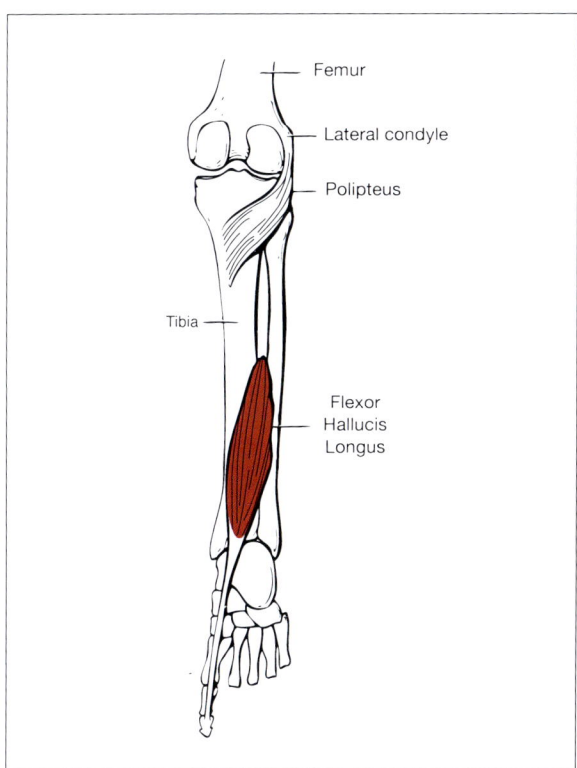

Flexor Hallucis Longus

Origin: distal two-thirds of posterior fibula; interosseous membrane; adjacent intermuscular septa and fascia.

Insertion: plantar surface of distal phalanx of big toe.

Innervation: tibial (L5-S2).

Action: flexes great toe; aids in plantarflexing the foot; gives medial ankle stability.

Chapman's reflexes
Anterior: inferior pubic bone
Posterior: L5/PSIS

Neurovascular point
frontal bone eminences

Nutrition
raw bone concentrate

Acupuncture meridian association
circulation sex

FLEXOR HALLUCIS LONGUS

Test

Position
Supine.

Test
Patient uses fingers to hold toes 2 through 5 in extension while examiner stabilizes the proximal phalanx of the great toe.

With the fingertip of the other hand, examiner contacts the plantar surface of the great toe and directs pressure toward extension.

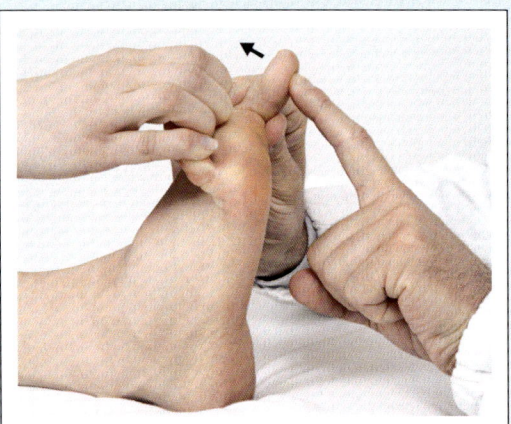

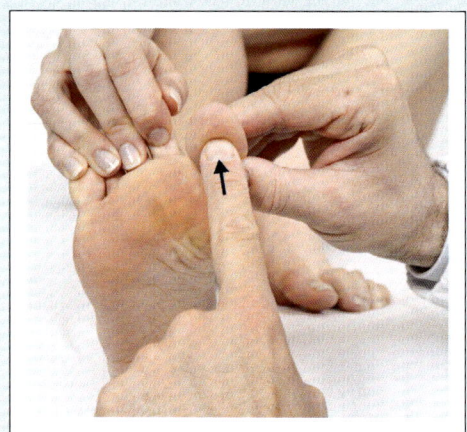

Alternate Test

Position
Supine.

Test
Patient holds foot midway between dorsiflexion and plantarflexion and keeps toes 2 through 5 in neutral position. Examiner stabilizes the proximal phalanx of the great toe in the web of his thumb and index fingers, while simultaneously positioning the same index finger along the plantar surfaces of toes 2 through 5 in order to prevent flexion. With a finger tip of the other hand, contact is made at the plantar surface of the distal phalanx of the great toe and pressure is directed toward extension.

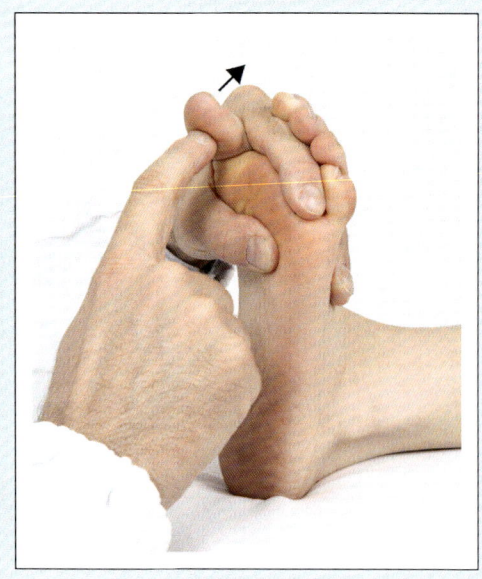

GASTROCNEMEUS

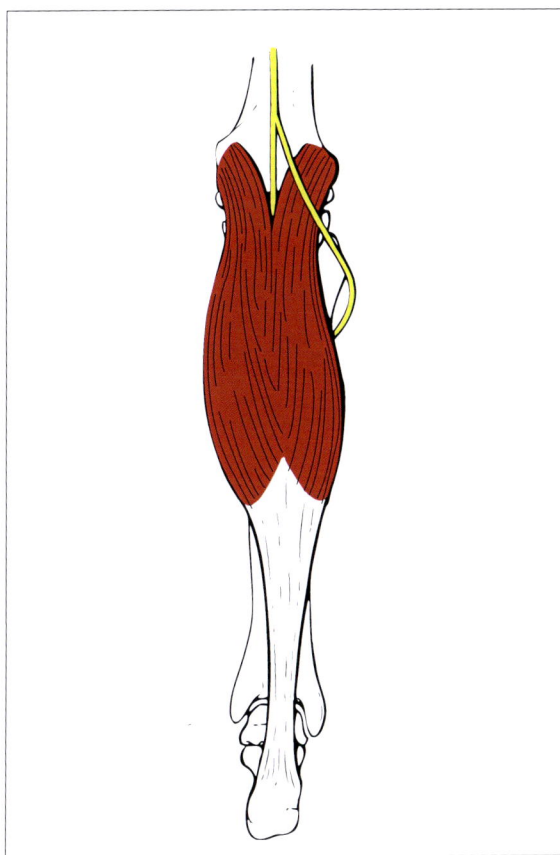

Gastrocnemeus
Origin lateral head: lateral aspect of lateral condyle of femur; posterior surface of knee joint.
Origin medial head: medial condyle and adjacent part of femur; capsule of knee joint.
Insertion: posterior surface of calcaneus via achilles tendon.
Innervation: tibial (L4-S2).
Action: plantarflexes foot; raises heel during walking; flexes knee joint.

Chapman's reflexes
Anterior: 1 inch lateral and 2 inches superior to umbillicus
Posterior: T11 and T12

Neurovascular point
lambda

Nutrition
adrenal substance; vitamin C; pantothenic acid; niacinamide; wheat germ oil; DHEA; adaptogens

Acupuncture meridian association
circulation sex (pericardium)

Common subluxations
L4-S2

Meric TS line
T9

Associated point
T4 and T5 (circulation sex)

Visceral association
adrenals

CLINICAL*

- important in "take off" phase of walking or running
- difficulty standing up on tip toes
- works with soleus
- any knee problems
- recurrent calcaneus subluxations
- cramps or "charley horses" at night (calcium metabolism)
- adrenals

*Courtesy of Drs. Walter Schmitt and Kerry McCord Quintessential Applications: A(K) Clinical Protocol (QA)

GASTROCNEMEUS

POSTURE

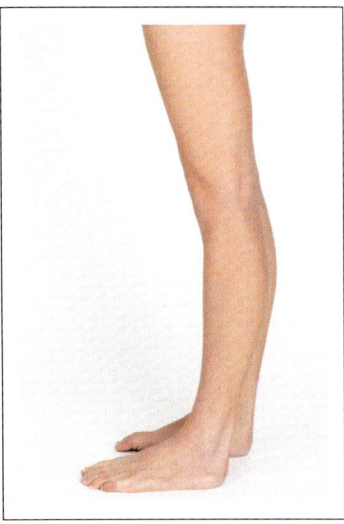

Hyperextended knee.

Test 1

Position
Supine.

Test
With teeth lightly clenched, supine patient flexes leg to 110 degrees and femur to 40 degrees. The foot is then either externally or internally rotated, depending on which head is being tested: internal rotation for medial head and vice versa. Examiner stands at the foot of the table and places one hand over the knee while the other hand grasps the posterior calcaneus. Force is applied through both hands simultaneously toward femur and leg extension.

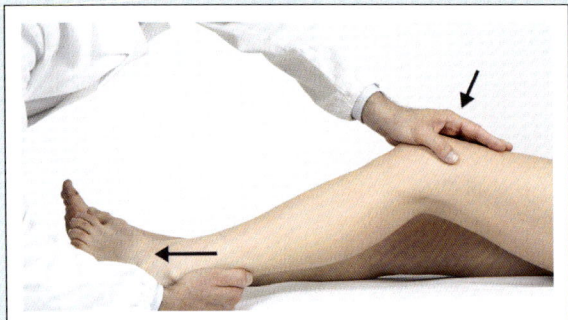
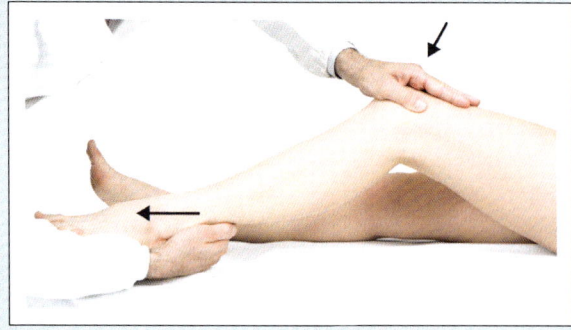

GASTROCNEMEUS

Test 2 Medial Head of Gastrocnemeus

Position
Prone.

Test
With teeth lightly clenched, patient flexes leg to about 30 degrees, and maximally rotates foot and leg internally. Examiner stands on side to be tested, contacts the postero-medial, distal leg and directs pressure toward leg extension. The vector of test pressure is away from the midline (down and out).

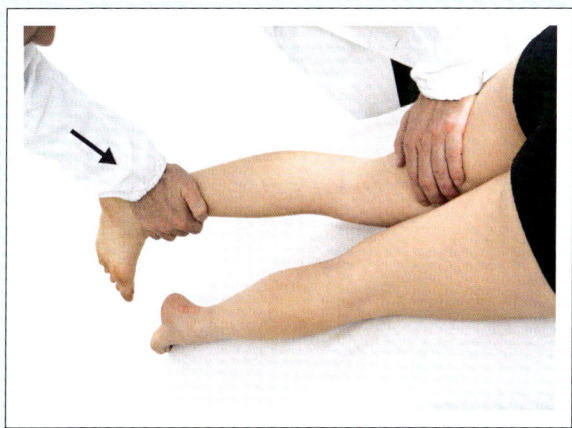

Test 2 Lateral Head of Gastrocnemeus

Position
Prone.

Test
Patient lightly clenches teeth, flexes leg to about 30 degrees, and maximally rotates foot and leg externally. Examiner stands on side to be tested, contacts the postero-lateral distal leg, and directs pressure toward leg extension. The vector of test pressure is toward the midline (down and in).

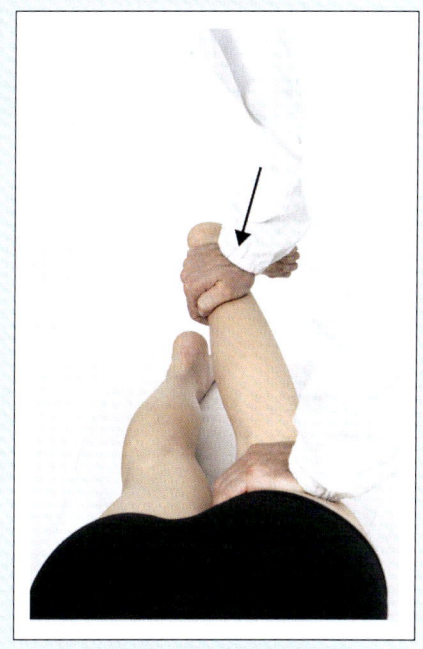

GASTROCNEMEUS

Test 3 Medial Head of Gastrocnemeus

Position
Prone.

Test
Patient lightly clenches teeth, fully flexes leg, and maximally rotates foot and leg internally. Examiner contacts the postero-medial distal leg, and directs pressure toward leg extension. The vector of test pressure is away from the midline (up and out).

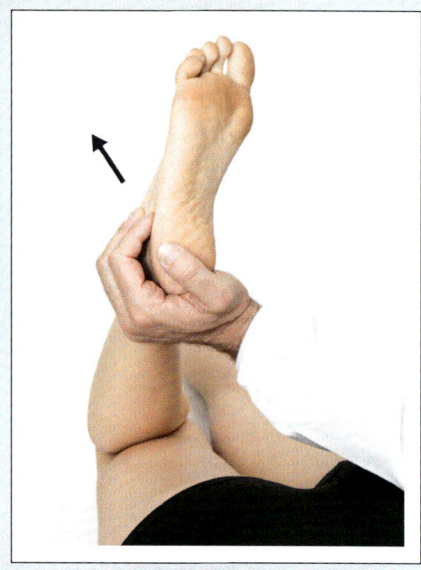

Test 3 Lateral Head of Gastrocnemeus

Position
Prone.

Test
Patient lightly clenches teeth, fully flexes leg, and maximally rotates foot and leg externally. Examiner contacts the postero-lateral, distal leg, and directs pressure toward leg extension. The vector of test pressure is toward the midline (up and in).

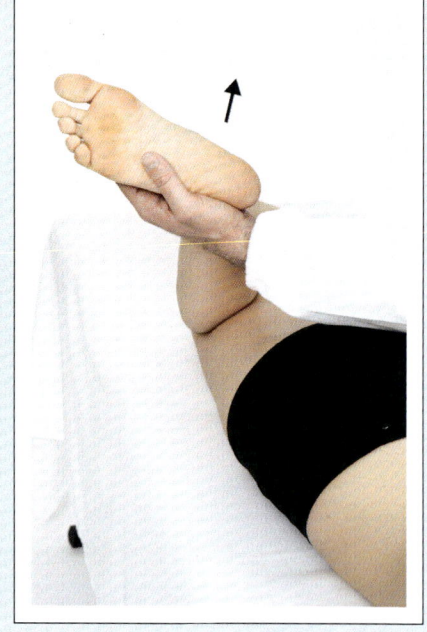

GLUTEUS MAXIMUS

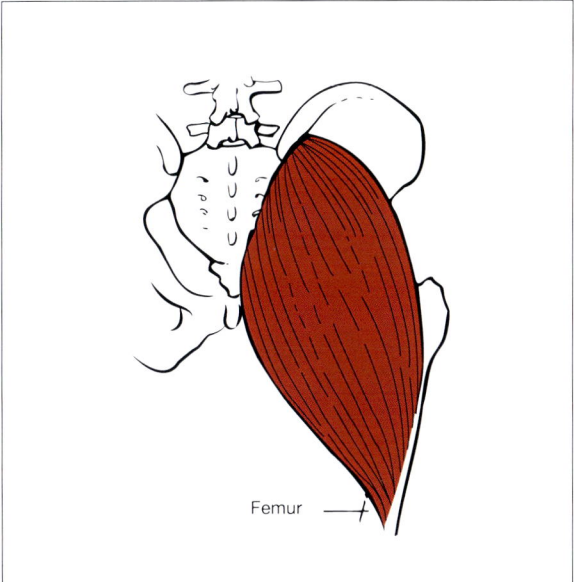
Femur

Gluteus Maximus
Origin: external surface of ala of ilium including iliac crest, tendon of sacrospinalis, dorsal surface of sacrum and coccyx, and sacrotuberous ligament.
Insertion: inferior gluteal (L4-S2).
Innervation: gluteal tuberosity of femur; iliotibial tract of fascia lata.
Action: extends femur and assists in its external rotation; raises trunk from bent forward position.

Chapman's reflexes
Anterior: lateral thigh (posterior to and overlapping TFL reflex)
Posterior: L5/PSIS

Neurovascular point
on lambdoidal suture midway between lambda and asterion

Nutrition
vitamin E; male or female organ substances

Acupuncture meridian association
circulation sex

Common subluxations
L4, L5 and sacrum

Meric TS line
L3

Associated point
T4 and T5 (circulation sex)

Visceral association
reproductive organs/glands

CLINICAL*

- trunk lurches backward at heel-strike phase of gait
- low back pain due to origin and insertion injury from trauma
- difficulty or back pain going up stairs
- bilateral weakness
- hyperlordosis (with abdominals)
- bilateral weakness
- upper cervical fixation
- uterus
- prostate
- lateral knee problems

*Courtesy of Drs. Walter Schmitt and Kerry McCord
Quintessential Applications: A(K) Clinical Protocol (QA)

GLUTEUS MAXIMUS

POSTURE

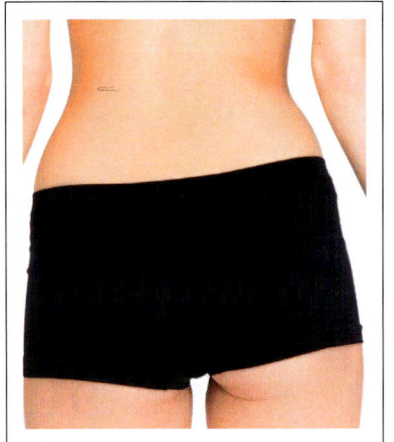

Unilateral weakness: high ipsilateral hip with anterior rotation of pelvis.

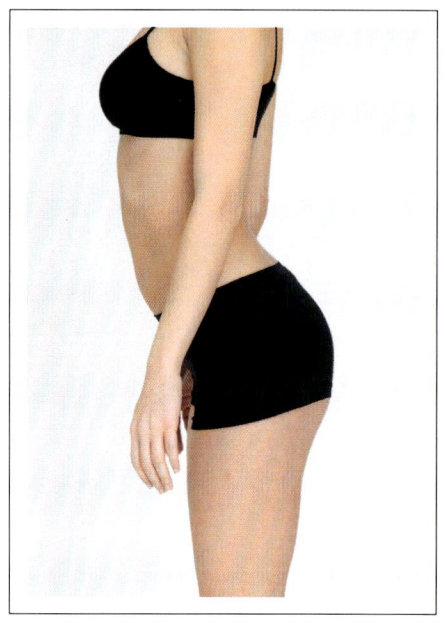

Bilateral weakness: hyperlordotic lumbar spine.

Test

Position
Prone.

Test
Patient flexes knee to 90 degrees then maximally extends femur. Examiner stands on side being tested and stabilizes with one hand over contralateral posterior iliac crest, while the other hand (or fist) contacts the posterior surface of the distal femur and directs pressure toward flexion.

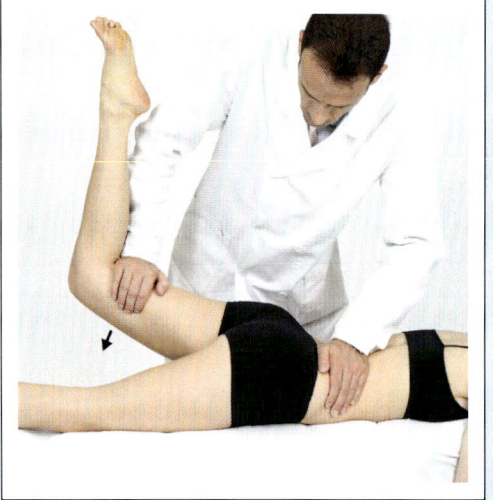 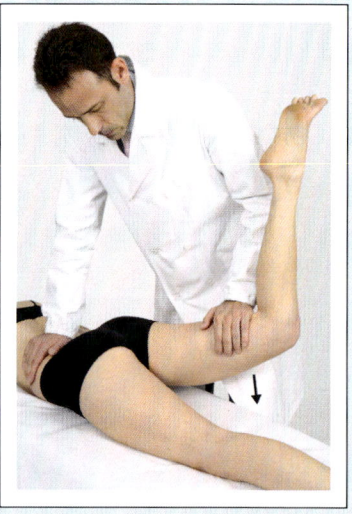

GLUTEUS MAXIMUS

Common errors

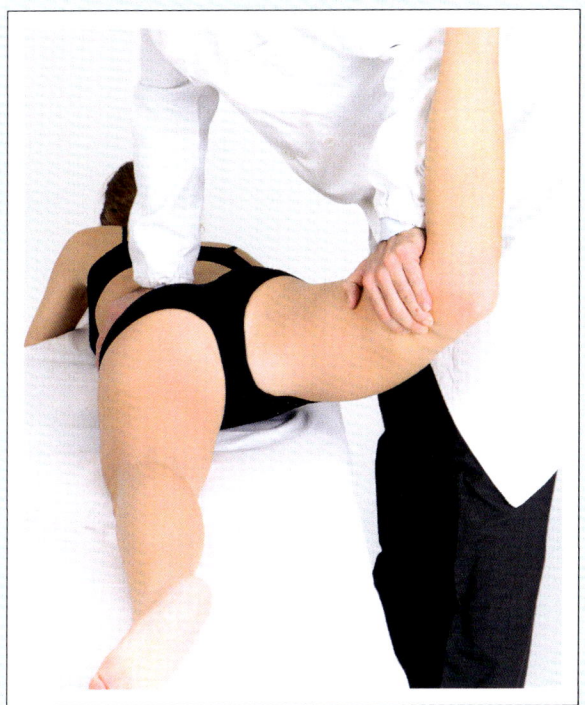

Abduction of femur in starting position.

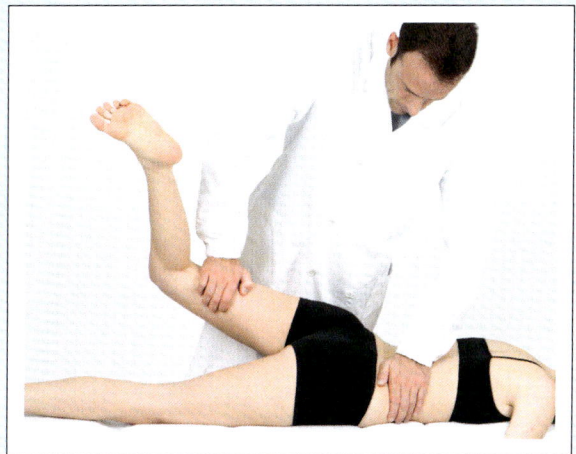

Pelvic or thigh external rotation.

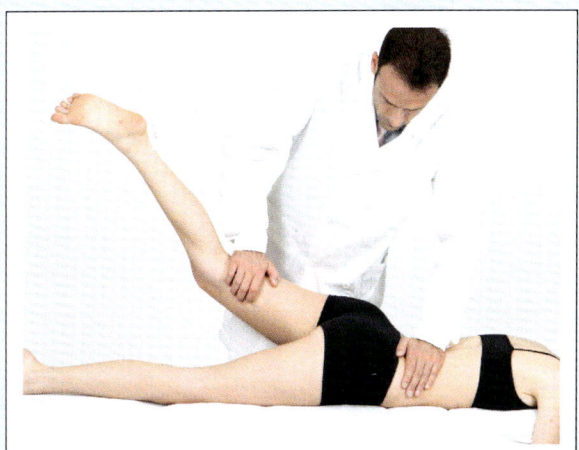

Knee extension.

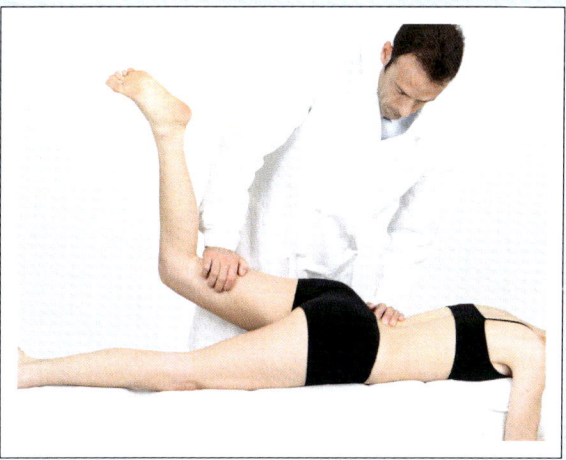

Examiner stabilizes ipsilaterally.

GLUTEUS MEDIUS
GLUTEUS MINIMUS

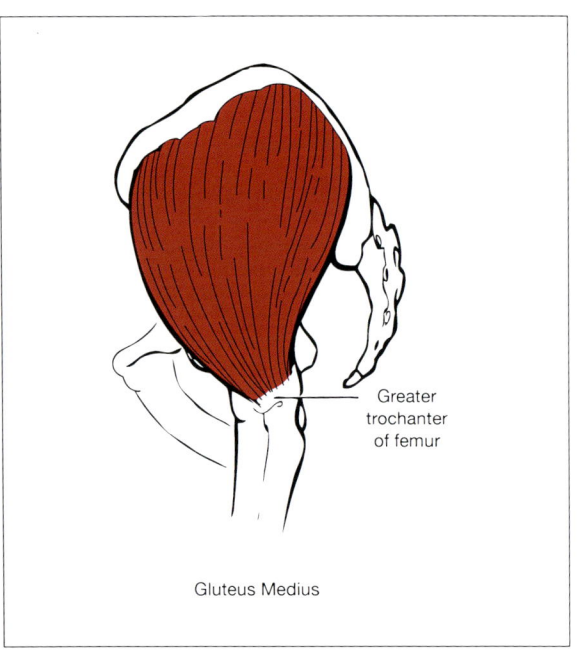
Gluteus Medius — Greater trochanter of femur

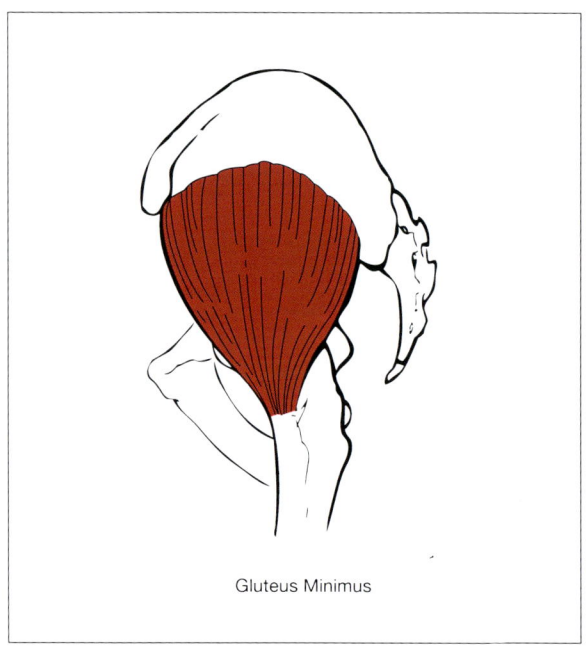
Gluteus Minimus

Gluteus medius and minimus are tested as a unit.

Gluteus Medius
Origin: external surface of the ilium between the iliac crest and the posterior gluteal line above, and the anterior gluteal line below; the gluteal aponeurosis.
Insertion: greater trochanter.
Innervation: superior gluteal (L4-S1).
Action: abducts and internally rotates femur; stabilizes pelvis; aids in early hip flexion.

Gluteus Minimus
Origin: external surface of ilium between anterior and inferior gluteal lines and margin of greater sciatic notch.
Insertion: greater trochanter.
Innervation: superior gluteal (L4-S1).
Action: abducts thigh and rotates it internally; assists gluteus medius in most functions.

CLINICAL*

- trunk lurches toward weak side during stance phase of gait
- hip/greater trochanter pain
- low back pain
- prostate
- uterus

*Courtesy of Drs. Walter Schmitt and Kerry McCord Quintessential Applications: A(K) Clinical Protocol (QA)

GLUTEUS MEDIUS AND GLUTEUS MINIMUS

Chapman's reflexes
Anterior: pubic bone
Posterior: L5/PSIS

Neurovascular point
on parietal eminence, posterior aspect

Nutrition
vitamin E;
male or female organ substances

Meric TS line
L5

Acupuncture meridian association
circulation sex

Common subluxations
L4, L5 and sacrum

Associated point
T4 and T5 (circulation sex)

Visceral association
reproductive organs/glands

Test 1

Position
Side-lying.

Test
Patient lies on the non-tested side and flexes the knee and hip in contact with the table both to approximately 45 degrees in order to create stability. Examiner stands behind the patient and further stabilizes with one hand on the flank. With the knee of the leg being tested locked in extension, and the femur in 10 to 20 degrees of extension, patient fully abducts femur. Examiner contacts distal, lateral femur (or the proximal leg, depending on leverage needed) and directs pressure toward adduction and slight flexion.

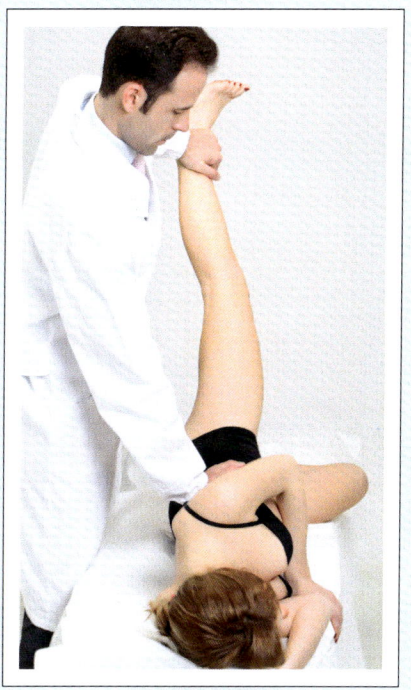
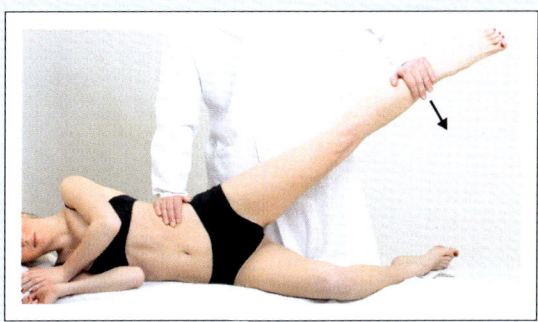

GLUTEUS MEDIUS AND GLUTEUS MINIMUS

Test 2

Position
Supine.

Test
Patient lightly clenches teeth then maximally abducts, slightly externally rotates, and extends the femur to about 10 to 20 degrees. Examiner stabilizes the non-tested leg with one hand, while the other contacts the lateral, distal leg on the side being tested, and uses it as a lever to impart pressure toward adduction, slight flexion, and slight internal rotation of the femur.

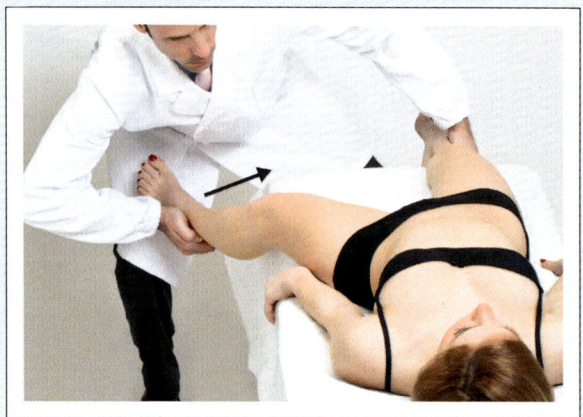

Common errors

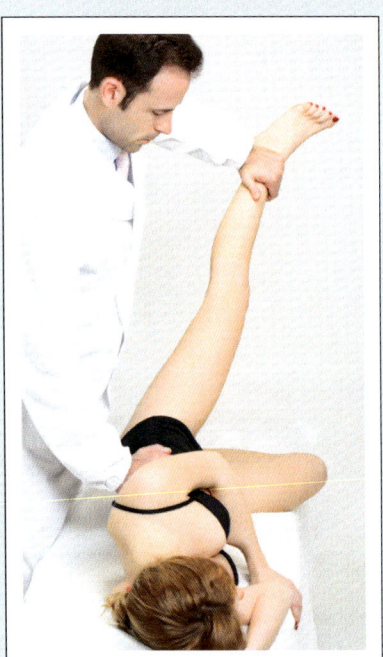

Too much femur flexion.

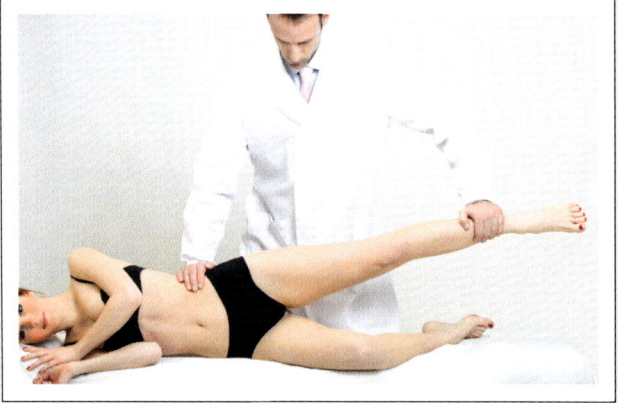

Not enough femur abduction.

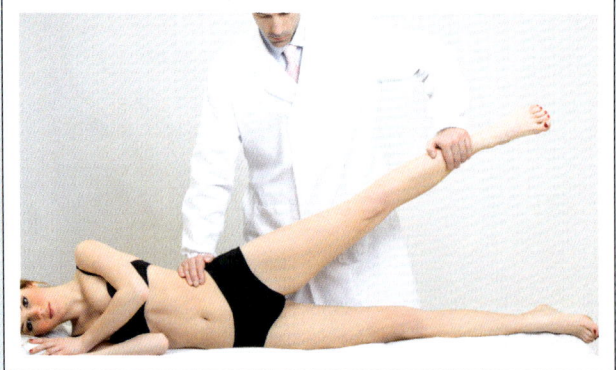

Non-tested, stabilizing leg not bent.

GRACILIS

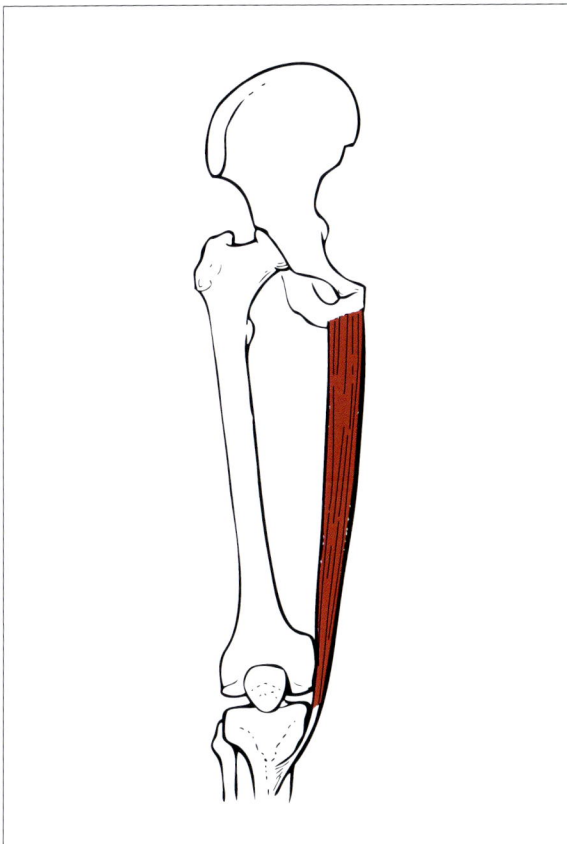

Gracilis
Origin: body and inferior ramus of pubis.

Insertion: pes anserinus superior part of medial surface of tibia.

Innervation: obturator (L2-L4).

Action: adducts femur; flexes and internally rotates femur and tibia.

Chapman's reflexes
Anterior: 1 inch lateral and 2 inches superior to umbillicus
Posterior: T11 and T12

Neurovascular point
lambda

Nutrition
adrenal substance; vitamin C; pantothenic acid; niacinamide; wheat germ oil; DHEA; adaptogens.

Acupuncture meridian association
circulation sex (pericardium)

Common subluxations
L2, L3 and L4

Meric TS line
T9

Associated point
T4 and T5 (circulation sex)

Visceral association
adrenals

CLINICAL*

- any knee problems
- medial meniscus injury
- tripod muscle: knee and pelvic stabilization
- category 2 posterior ilium (UoMS)
- adrenals

*Courtesy of Drs. Walter Schmitt and Kerry McCord
Quintessential Applications: A(K) Clinical Protocol (QA)

GRACILIS

POSTURE

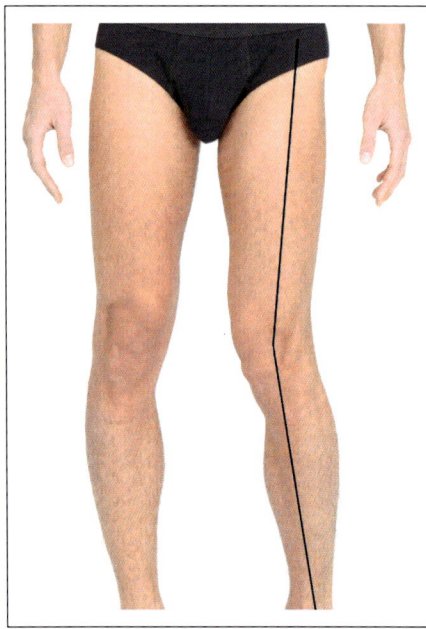

Genu valgus ("knock knees"); pelvic posterior rotation on weak side.

Test 1

Position
Prone.

Test
With teeth lightly clenched, patient plantarflexes foot, flexes leg to approximately 45 degrees, internally rotates and slightly abducts femur to about 30 to 40 degrees. Examiner stands on the side being tested and elevates the distal femur to approximately 30 degrees of extension. This can be done by wedging a fist between the anterior, distal thigh and the table. The other hand contacts the posterior, distal leg and directs pressure toward extension, away from the midline to impart pressure toward internal rotation of the femur.

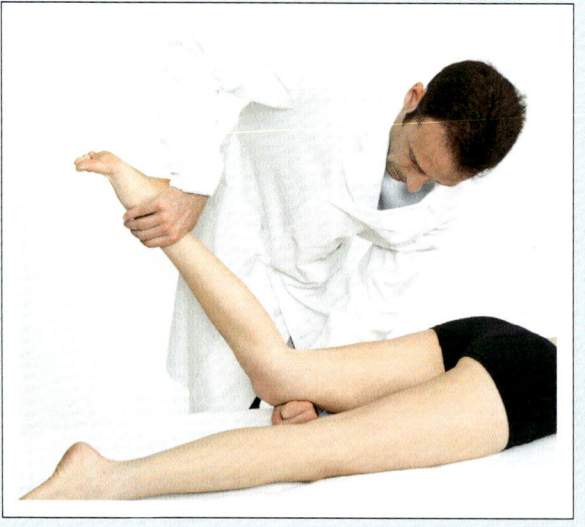

GRACILIS

Test 2

Position
Supine.

Test
With teeth lightly clenched, patient locks knee into extension and maximally internally rotates femur. Examiner uses one hand to stabilize the contralateral leg, while the other hand contacts the medial surface of the ipsilateral, distal leg and uses it as a lever to impart pressure toward abduction, and slight flexion of the femur (out and up).

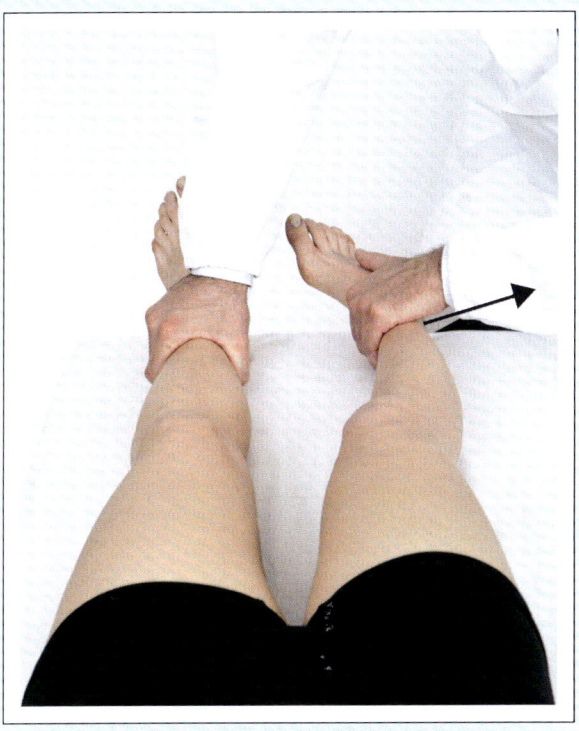

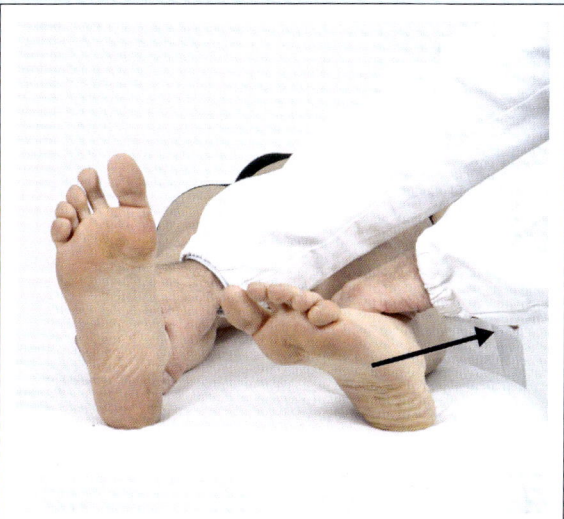

HAMSTRINGS

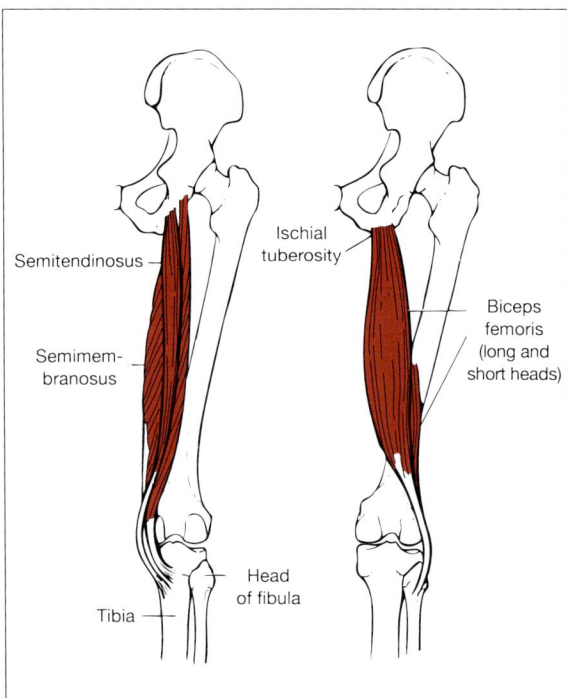

The hamstrings muscles are divided into medial hamstrings (semitendinosus and semimembranosus) and lateral hamstrings (biceps femoris).

Semitendinosus and Semimembranosus (Medial Hamstrings)

Origin: ischial tuberosity.

Insertion: medial surface of proximal tibia; posterior portion of medial condyle of tibia (pes anserinus).

Innervation: sciatic (tibial branch L4-S2).

Action: flexes and internally rotates the leg (knee joint); extends, adducts, and internally rotates femur.

Biceps Femoris (Lateral Hamstrings)

Origin long head: ischial tuberosity and sacrotuberous ligament.

Origin short head: lateral lip of linea aspera; lateral supracondyle of femur; lateral intermuscular septum.

Insertion: lateral surface of head of fibula; lateral condyle of tibia; deep fascia on lateral surface of leg.

Innervation long head: sciatic (tibial branch L5-S3).

Innervation short head: sciatic (peroneal branch L5-S2).

Action: flexes and externally rotates leg (knee joint); extends, adducts and externally rotates femur.

CLINICAL*

- lateral knee pain with weak lateral hamstrings
- medial knee pain with weak medial hamstrings
- anterior pelvic subluxation
- "pulled hamstrings"
- rectum
- hemorrhoids

*Courtesy of Drs. Walter Schmitt and Kerry McCord
Quintessential Applications: A(K) Clinical Protocol (QA)

HAMSTRINGS

The following applies to the hamstrings as a group:

Chapman's reflexes
Anterior: over lesser trochanter
Posterior: PSIS/L5

Neurovascular point
1 inch above lambda

Nutrition
vitamin E; if cramping exists, calcium, including HCl

Acupuncture meridian association
large intestine

Common subluxations
L4-S2

Meric TS line
L1

Associated point
L4 and L5 (large intestine)

Visceral association
rectum

POSTURE

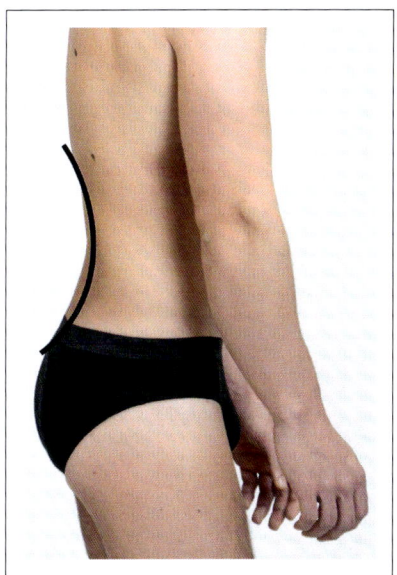

Hamstrings as a group: anterior pelvic tilt, lumbar hyperlordosis.

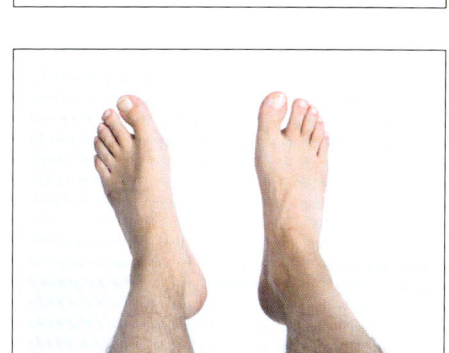

Medial Hamstrings: external foot rotation.

Lateral Hamstrings: internal foot rotation

HAMSTRINGS

Test for Hamstrings (group test)

Position
Best tested prone, can also be tested supine.

Test
Patient lightly clenches teeth, flexes knee (70-80 degrees) and plantarflexes foot.
Examiner stands on the side being tested and stabilizes with one hand over the belly of the hamstrings to prevent cramping, while the other hand contacts the distal, posterior leg and directs pressure toward leg extension.

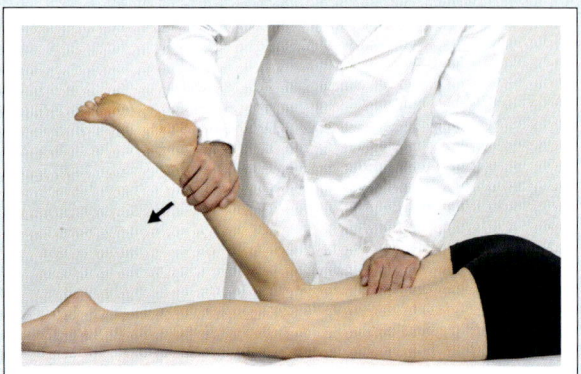

Test for Medial Hamstrings

Position
Best tested prone, can also be tested supine.

Test
Patient lightly clenches teeth, flexes knee (70-80 degrees), plantarflexes foot, and internally rotates thigh.
Examiner stands on the side being tested and stabilizes with one hand over the belly of the hamstrings to prevent cramping, while the other hand contacts the distal, posterior leg and directs pressure toward leg extension, away from the midline, in order to impart simultaneous pressure toward internal rotation of the femur.

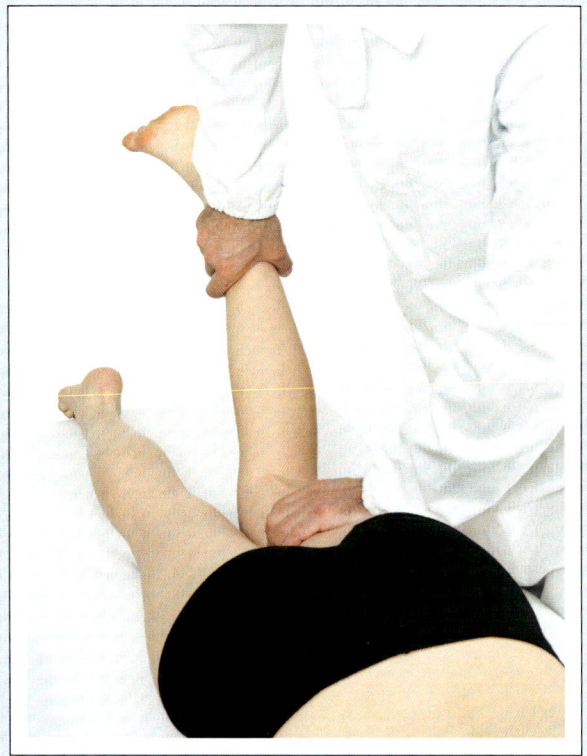

HAMSTRINGS

Test for Lateral Hamstrings

Position
Best tested prone, can also be tested supine.

Test
Patient lightly clenches teeth, flexes knee (70-80 degrees), plantarflexes foot, and externally rotates thigh. Examiner stands on the side being tested and stabilizes with one hand over the belly of the hamstrings to prevent cramping, while the other hand contacts the distal, posterior leg and directs pressure toward leg extension, toward the midline, in order to impart simultaneous pressure toward external rotation of the femur.

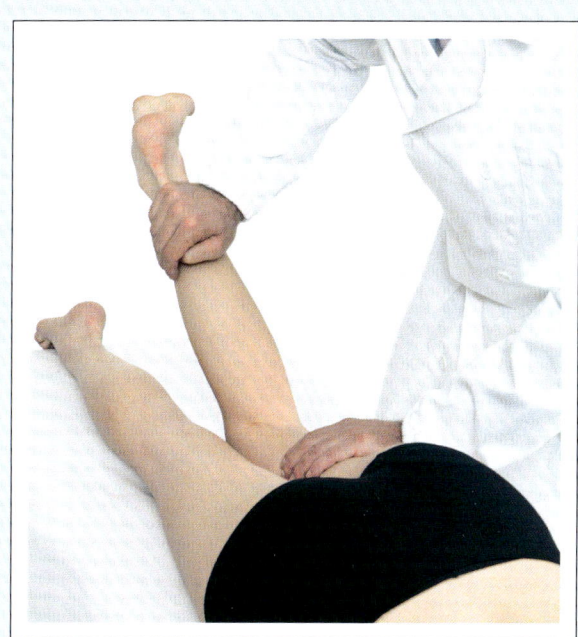

Common errors

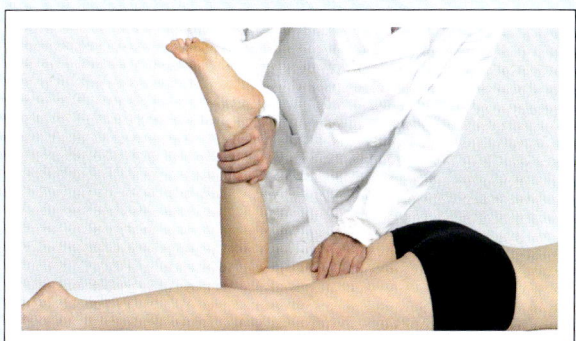

Too much flexion of knee.

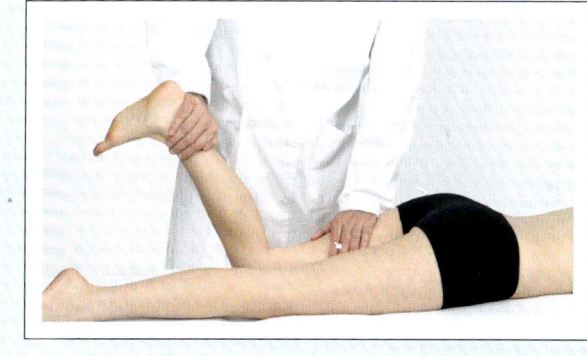

Ankle is allowed to dorsiflex.

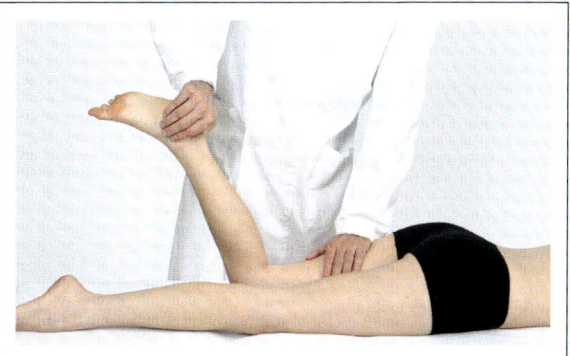

Pressure is on calcaneus instead of distal leg.

ILIACUS

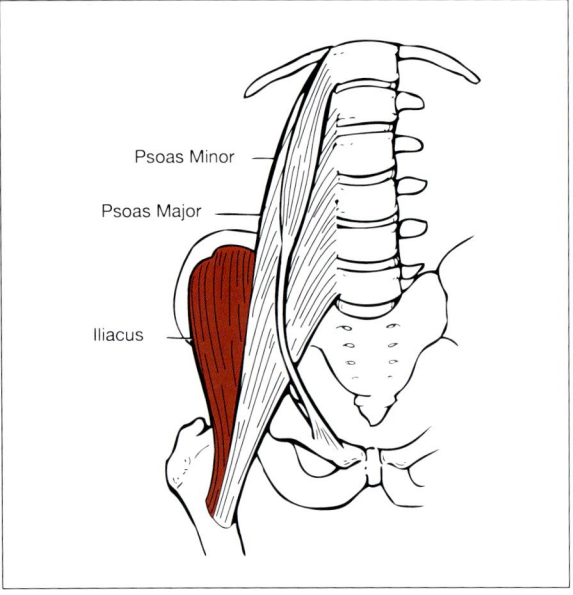

Iliacus
Origin: upper two-thirds of iliac fossa; internal border of iliac crest; anterior sacroiliac, lumbosacral and iliolumbar ligaments; ala of sacrum.

Insertion: lesser trochanter of femur.

Innervation: femoral (L1-L3).

Action: with psoas, flexes, abducts, and externally rotates femur.

Chapman's reflexes
Anterior: 1 inch lateral and 1 inch superior to umbillicus
Posterior: T12, L1

Neurovascular point
1-1/2 inch lateral to external occipital protuberance

Nutrition
vitamin A and E
kidney substance

Acupuncture meridian association
kidney

Common subluxations
sacral and pelvic

Associated point
L2 and L3 (kidney)

Visceral association
kidney (sometimes associated with ileocecal valve)

CLINICAL*

- low back pain
- supine: greater foot turn in on weak side
- ipsilateral foot pronation
- kidney problems including renalithiasis
- sacroiliac misalignments

*Courtesy of Drs. Walter Schmitt and Kerry McCord Quintessential Applications: A(K) Clinical Protocol (QA)

ILIACUS

POSTURE

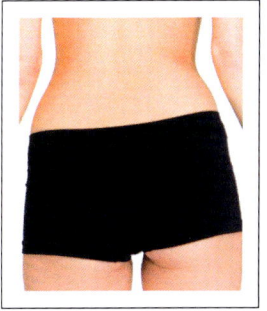
Pelvis elevated on weak side.

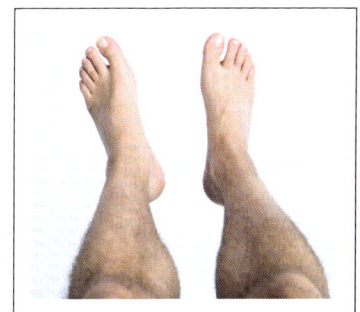
Toe turn in on weak side (best seen with patient supine).

Test

Position
Supine.

Test
The patient is positioned as in the test for iliopsoas but with more abduction and flexion of the femur: the knee is locked in extension, as the patient flexes, abducts, and externally rotates the femur. Examiner stabilizes with one hand over the contralateral anterior superior iliac spine, while the other hand contacts the antero-medial leg (or thigh depending how much leverage is needed) and directs pressure toward extension and abduction.

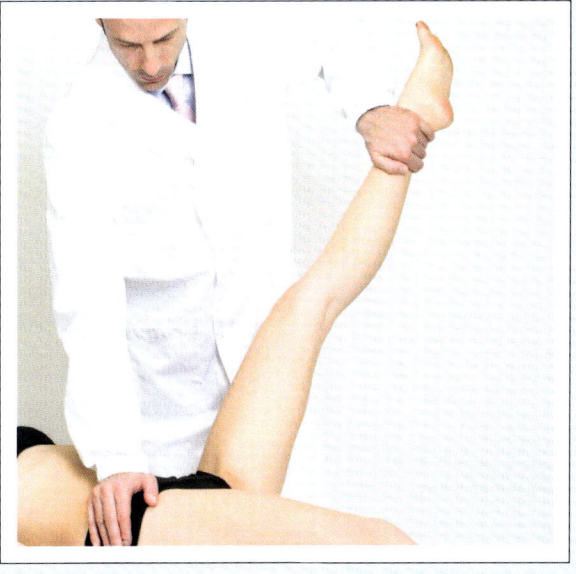
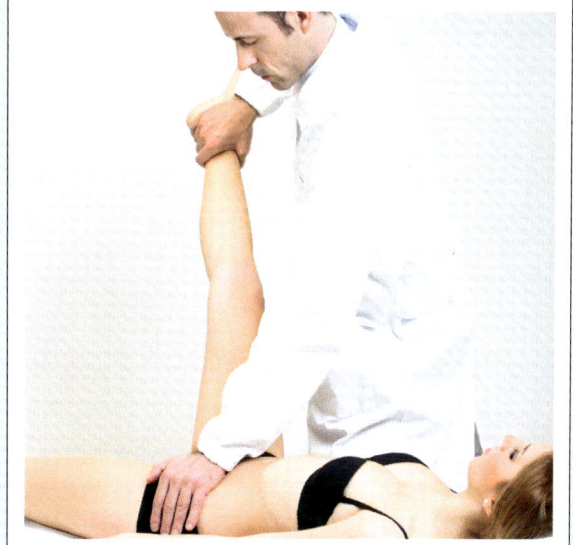

ILIOPSOAS
PSOAS MAJOR AND PSOAS MINOR

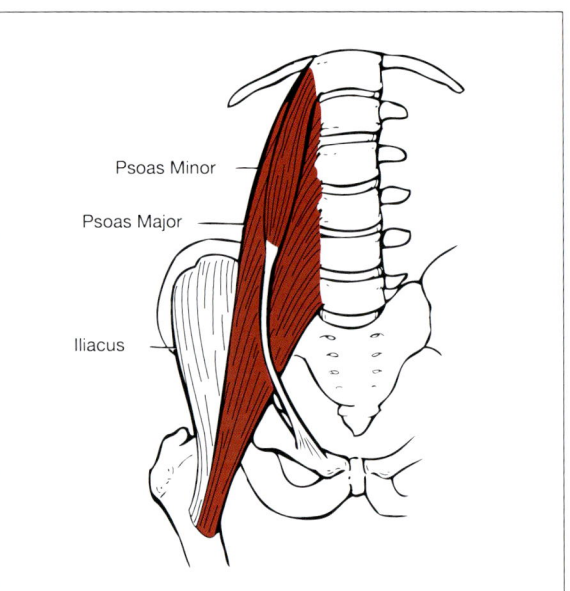

The term Iliopsoas refers to the combination of three muscles: psoas major, psoas minor, and iliacus. In muscle testing, psoas major and psoas minor are tested together.

Psoas major and Psoas minor
Origin: anterior surfaces of transverse processes, lateral borders of verterbral bodies and neighboring intervertebral discs of T12-L5.

Insertion: lesser trochanter of femur.

Innervation: lumbar plexus (L1-L4).

Action: flexion and external rotation of femur.

CLINICAL*

- low back pain
- lumbar scoliosis (concave on weak side)
- bilateral weakness creates flat or hypolordotic lumbar spine
- greater foot turn in on weak side, best seen with patient supine
- holds femur head in acetabulum (similar to supraspinatus function in glenohumeral joint), therefore hip pain when weak
- ipsilateral foot pronation
- kidney problems including renalithiasis

*Courtesy of Drs. Walter Schmitt and Kerry McCord
Quintessential Applications: A(K) Clinical Protocol (QA)

ILIOPSOAS PSOAS MAJOR AND PSOAS MINOR

Chapman's reflexes
Anterior: 1 inch lateral and 1 inch superior to umbillicus
Posterior: T12-L1

Neurovascular point
1-1/2 inch lateral to external occipital protuberance

Nutrition
vitamin A and E
kidney substance

Meric TS line T11 and T12

Acupuncture meridian association
kidney

Common subluxations
L1-L5

Associated point
L2 and L3 (kidney)

Visceral association
kidney

POSTURE

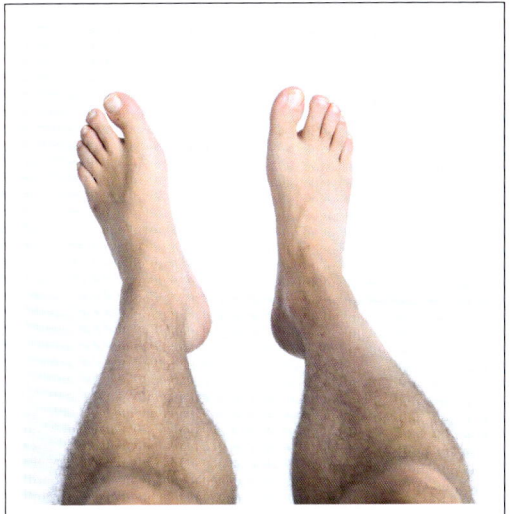

Toe turn in on weak side (best seen with patient supine).

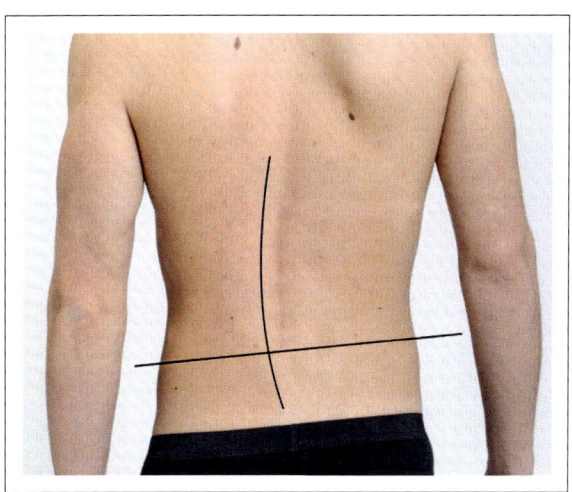

Pelvis elevated on weak side; lumbar vertebrae deviate away from weak side.

ILIOPSOAS PSOAS MAJOR AND PSOAS MINOR

Test

Position
Best tested supine, can also be performed seated.

Test
Keeping the knee locked in extension, patient flexes, abducts, and externally rotates the femur. Examiner stabilizes with one hand over the contralateral anterior superior iliac spine, while the other hand contacts the antero-medial leg (or thigh depending on how much leverage is needed) and directs pressure toward extension and slight abduction.

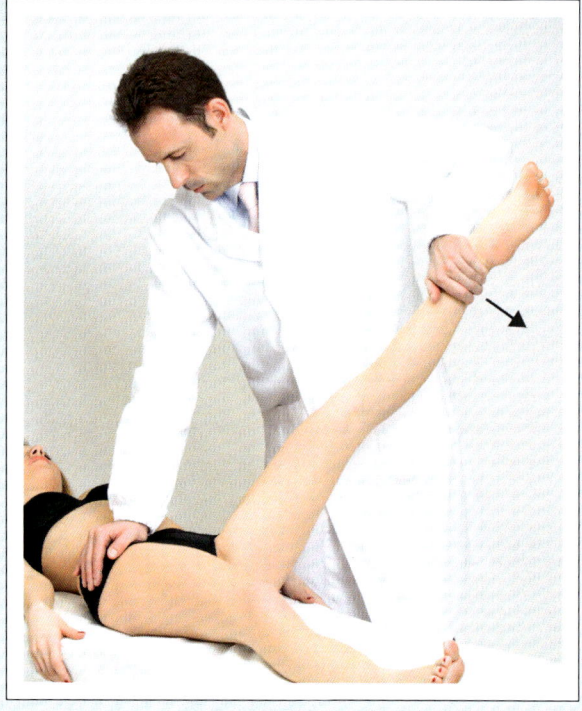

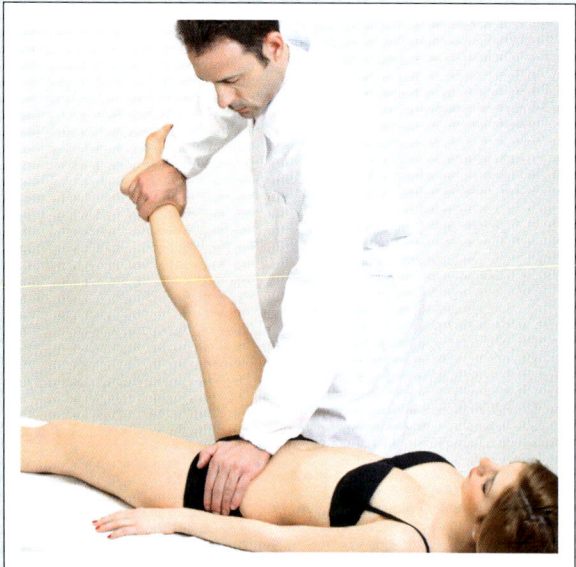

ILIOPSOAS PSOAS MAJOR AND PSOAS MINOR

Common errors — Iliacus and Iliopsoas.

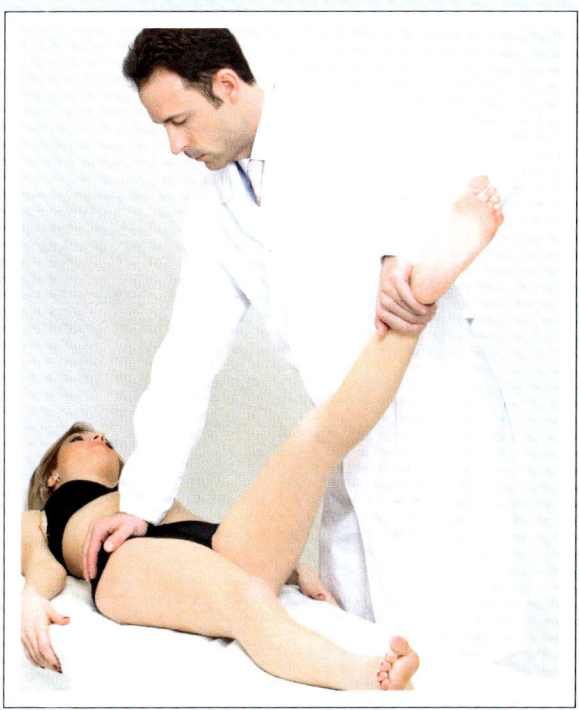

Wrong starting position: not enough femur abduction.

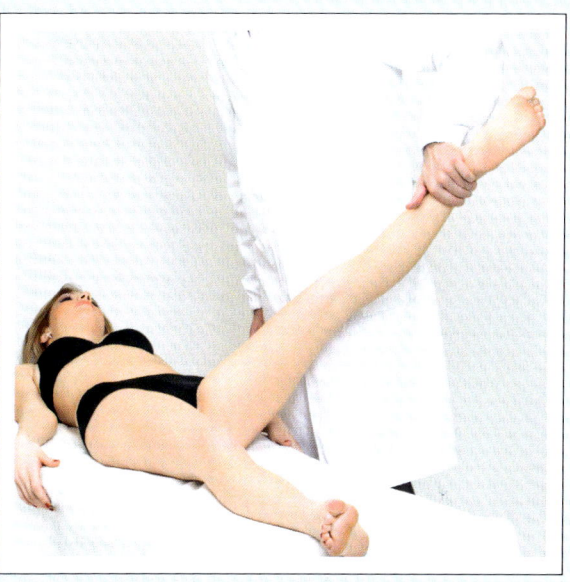

No stabilization.

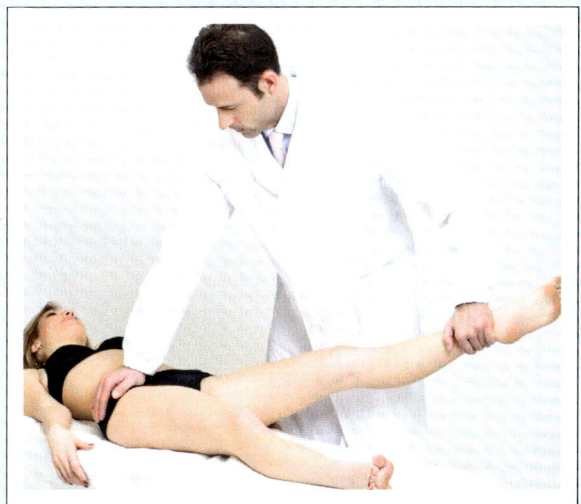

Not enough thigh flexion.

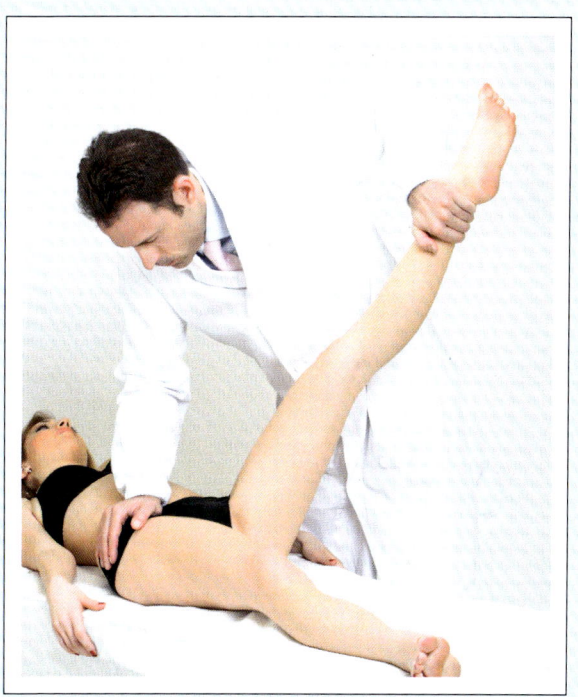

Examiner assumes bad posture.

INFRASPINATUS

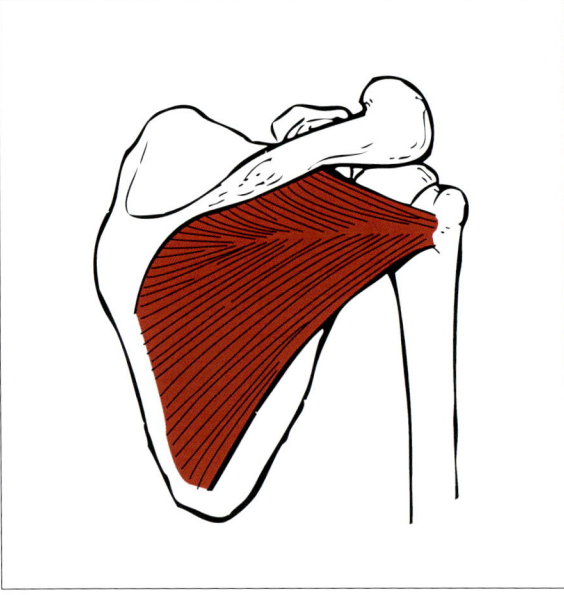

Infraspinatus
Origin: medial two-thirds of infraspinatus fossa of scapula.
Insertion: middle facet of greater tubercle of humerus and capsule of shoulder joint.
Innervation: suprascapular nerve (C5-C6).
Action: external rotation of humerus; assists in stabilization of head of humerus in glenoid cavity.

POSTURE

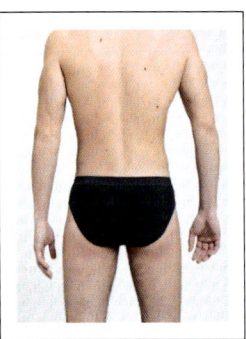

Arm, forearm, and hand hang in internal rotation (palm faces backward).

CLINICAL*

- difficulty with shoulder elevation
- difficulty reaching backward
- can't raise arm overhead with palm up
- difficulty playing tennis (backhand), golf, etc.
- origin and insertion injury in "rotator cuff syndrome"
- origin and insertion injury in scapular origin
- thymus

*Courtesy of Drs. Walter Schmitt and Kerry McCord
Quintessential Applications: A(K) Clinical Protocol (QA)

Chapman's reflexes
Anterior (only): right 5th intercostal space from mid-axillary line to mid-mammillary line

Neurovascular point
angle of Louis

Nutrition
thymus substance; immune system support substances

Acupuncture meridian association
triple heater

Common subluxations
C5 and C6

Associated point
L1 and L2 (triple warmer)

Visceral association
thymus

INFRASPINATUS

Test

Position
Seated, supine or prone.

Test
When seated or supine, patient lightly clenches teeth, then abducts humerus to 90 degrees and flexes forearm to 90 degrees. Examiner uses one hand to stabilize the lateral surface of the distal humerus, while the other contacts the distal, posterior forearm and uses it as a lever to direct pressure toward internal rotation of the humerus.

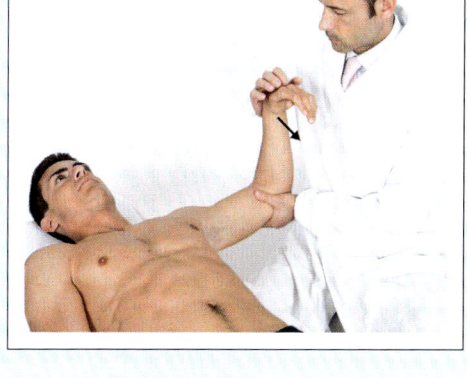

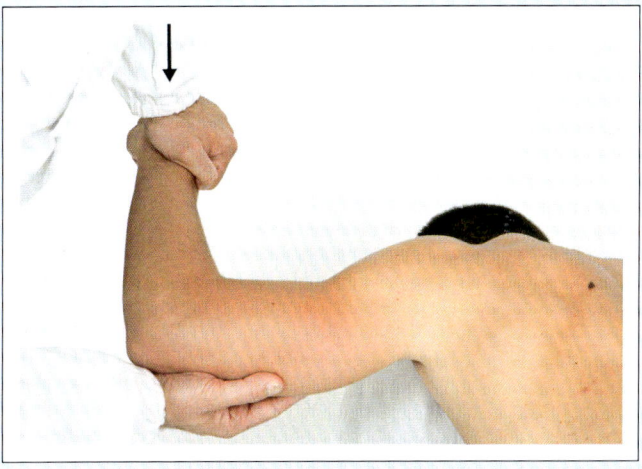

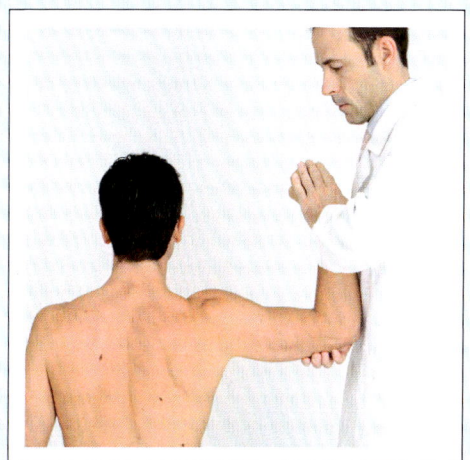

Common errors

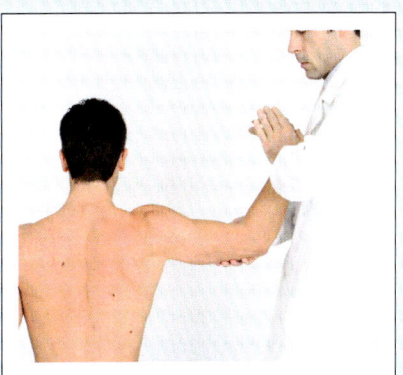

Excess forearm extension.

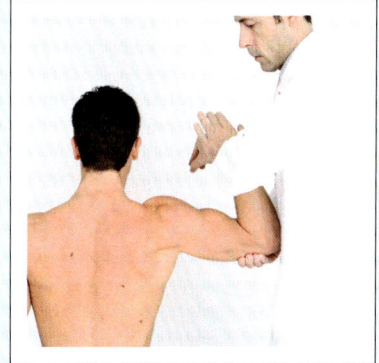

Excess forearm flexion.

LATISSIMUS DORSI

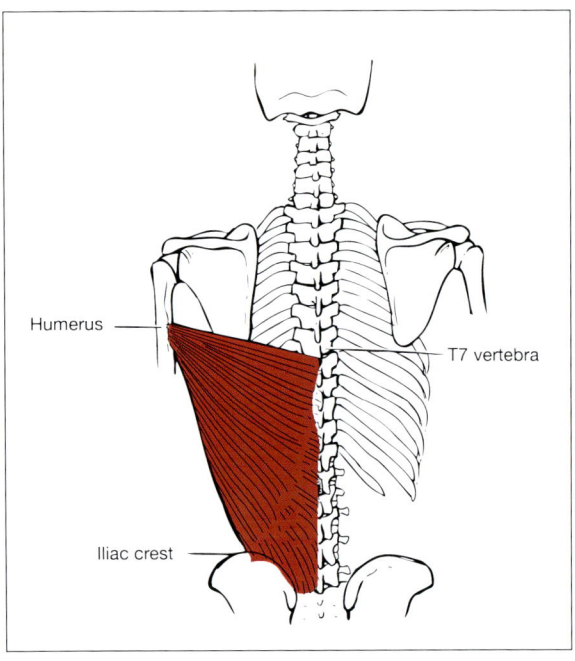

Latissimus Dorsi

Origin: thoracolumbar fascia; spinous processes of T6-T12 and L1-L5 vertebrae; sacrum; posterior iliac crest; inferior 3 or 4 posterior ribs; an attachment to the tip of the inferior angle of the scapula.

Insertion: floor of the intertubercular groove of humerus.

Innervation: thoracodorsal from brachial plexus (C6-C8).

Action: extension, adduction, and internal rotation of the humerus; draws the inferior angle of the scapula inferiorly and medially.

CLINICAL*

- upper trapezius tightness/difficulty and pain turning neck
- difficulty swimming or paddling a canoe
- holds shoulder down
- works with pectoralis major sternum, therefore pain and difficulty with ordinary pushing, parallel bars, or rings
- sacroiliac problems, especially during lifting
- on rare occasion, when tight can cause ipsilateral frozen shoulder
- pancreas: diabetes, hyperinsulism, blood-sugar handling problems

*Courtesy of Drs. Walter Schmitt and Kerry McCord
Quintessential Applications: A(K) Clinical Protocol (QA)

LATISSIMUS DORSI

Chapman's reflexes
Anterior: left 7th intercostal space
Posterior: left T7-T8

Neurovascular point
1 cm. above squamous suture just posterior to the external auditory meatus

Nutrition
betaine hydrochloride; pancreas concentrate of nucleoprotein extract; zinc; glucose regulation related substances (chromium, vanadium, etc.); vitamin A and vitamin F (EFA)

Acupuncture meridian association
spleen/pancreas

Meric TS line
T6

Common subluxations
C6, C7 and C8

Associated point
T11, T12 (spleen pancreas)

Visceral association
pancreas

POSTURE

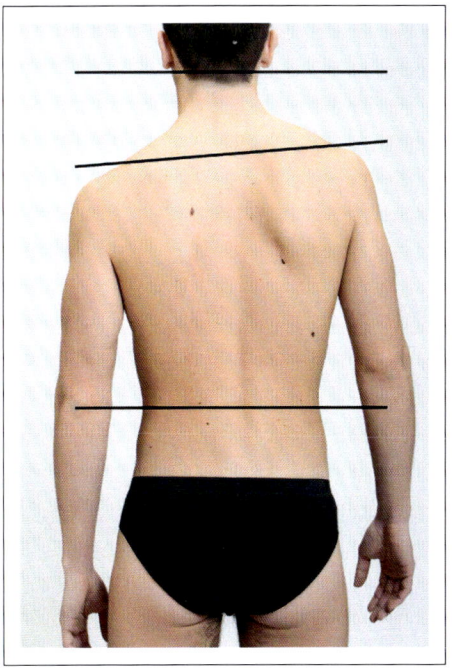

Shoulder is elevated and rolled forward with humerus in slight abduction on weak side.
Head will be level if other muscles are not involved.

LATISSIMUS DORSI

Test

Position
Seated, supine, prone, or standing.

Test
When seated, supine or standing, the patient gently clenches teeth, extends forearm, locking it at the elbow, then adducts and internally rotates humerus so that the anticubital fossa faces medially (thumb pointing toward buttocks).

Examiner contacts the lateral surface of the distal forearm (avoiding contact with pulse points) and uses the forearm as lever to direct pressure toward abduction and slight flexion of the humerus.

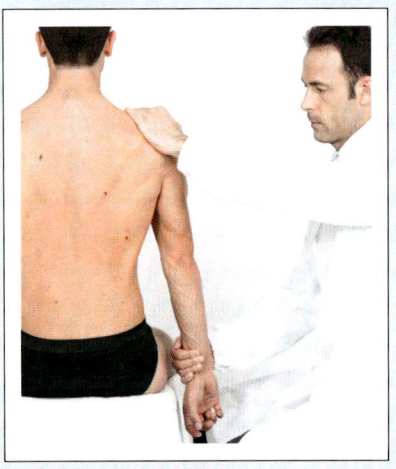
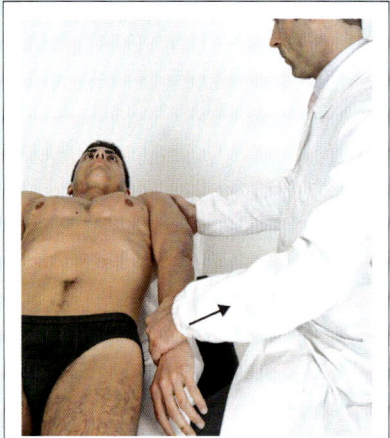
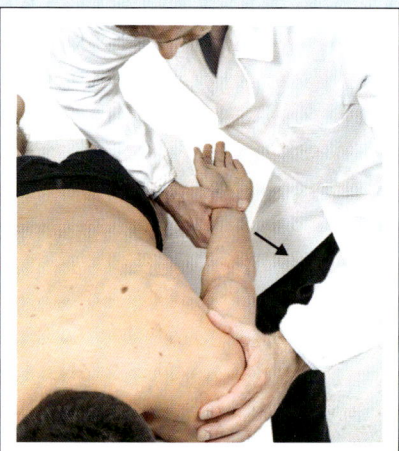

Common errors

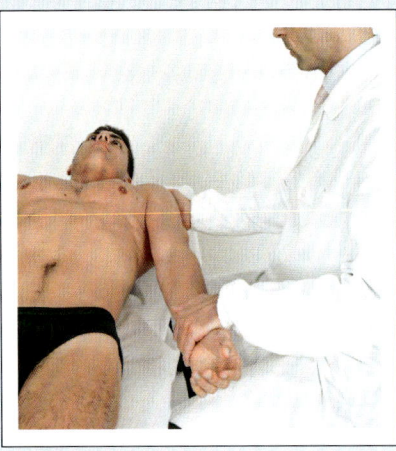

Humerus is allowed to laterally rotate.

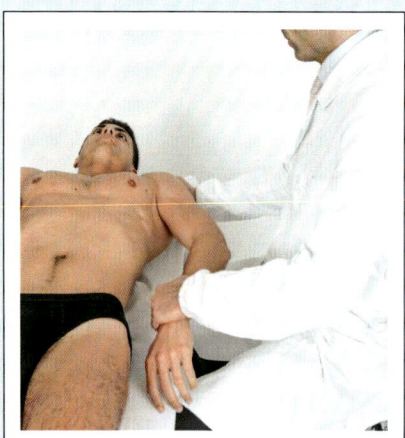

Elbow is allowed to bend.

LEVATOR SCAPULA

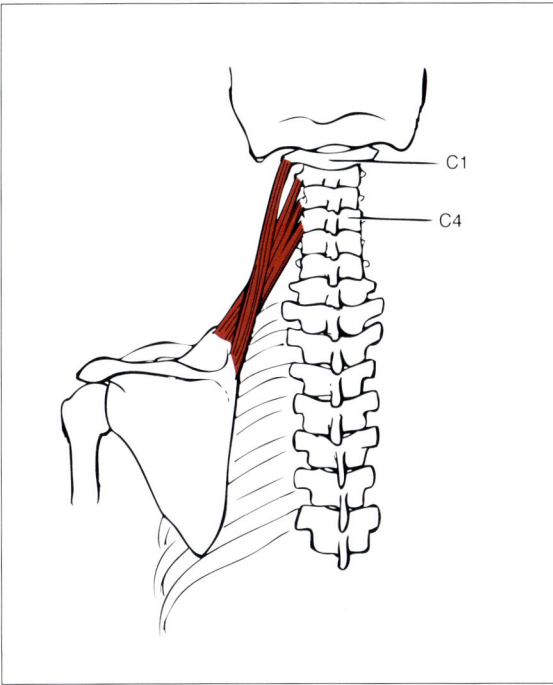

Levator Scapula
Origin: transverse processes of C1-C4 vertebrae.

Insertion: superior part of medial border of scapula.

Innervation: dorsal scapular (C3-C5).

Action: raises scapula to inferiorly rotate glenoid cavity; elevates and adducts scapula.

Chapman's reflexes
Anterior: 1st intercostal space peristernally
Posterior: belly of teres minor muscle

Neurovascular point
bregma

Nutrition
parathyroid substances

Acupuncture meridian association
lung

Common subluxations
cervical

Associated point
T3 and T4 lung

Visceral association
parathyroid

CLINICAL*

- pain in the origin and/or insertion
- pain in contralateral levator scapula
- pain in ipsilateral or contralateral upper trapezius
- patient awakens with "crick" in neck
- difficulty pain with lateral flexion and/or rotation
- whiplash injuries (origin/insertion)
- recurrent cervical subluxations
- parathyroid relationship
- general muscle tension and pain to palpation (pseudofibromyalgia)

*Courtesy of Drs. Walter Schmitt and Kerry McCord
Quintessential Applications: A(K) Clinical Protocol (QA)

LEVATOR SCAPULA

POSTURE

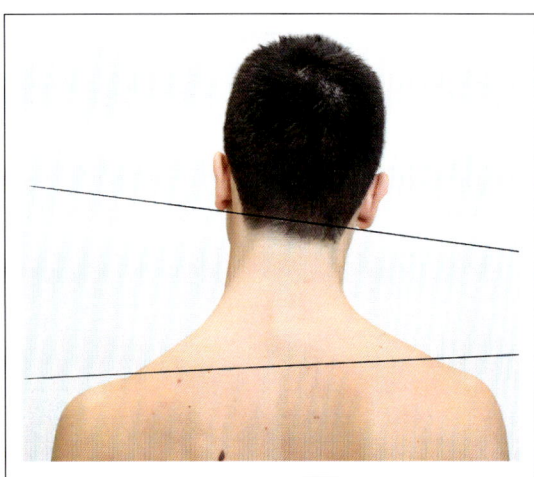

Occiput and shoulder separated on contralateral side of weakness.

Test

Position
Best tested seated.

Test
Seated patient gently clenches teeth then laterally flexes the thoracic spine toward the side being tested, keeping head and cervical spine vertical. This is done by dropping the ipsilateral shoulder as though trying to reach the table with elbow. The humerus is maintained in adduction and slight extension as examiner contacts the medial, distal portion to direct pressure toward abduction. During the test, examiner observes the superior angle of the scapula for inferior rotation, which would indicate a positive test.

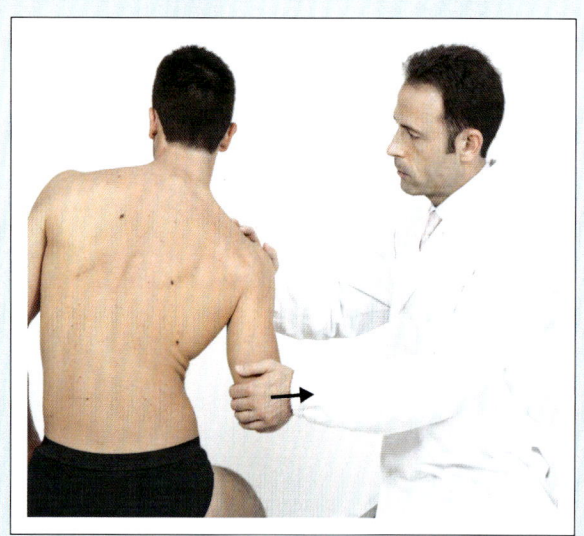

Common errors

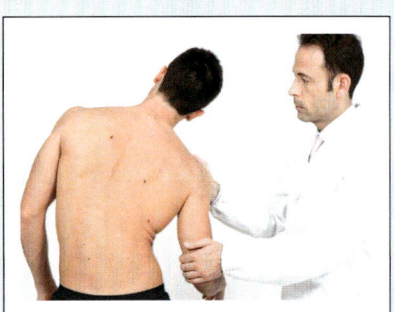

Head is allowed to tilt.

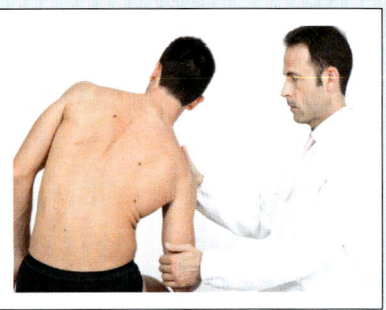

Excessive lateral flexion of the trunk.

MEDIAL NECK FLEXORS

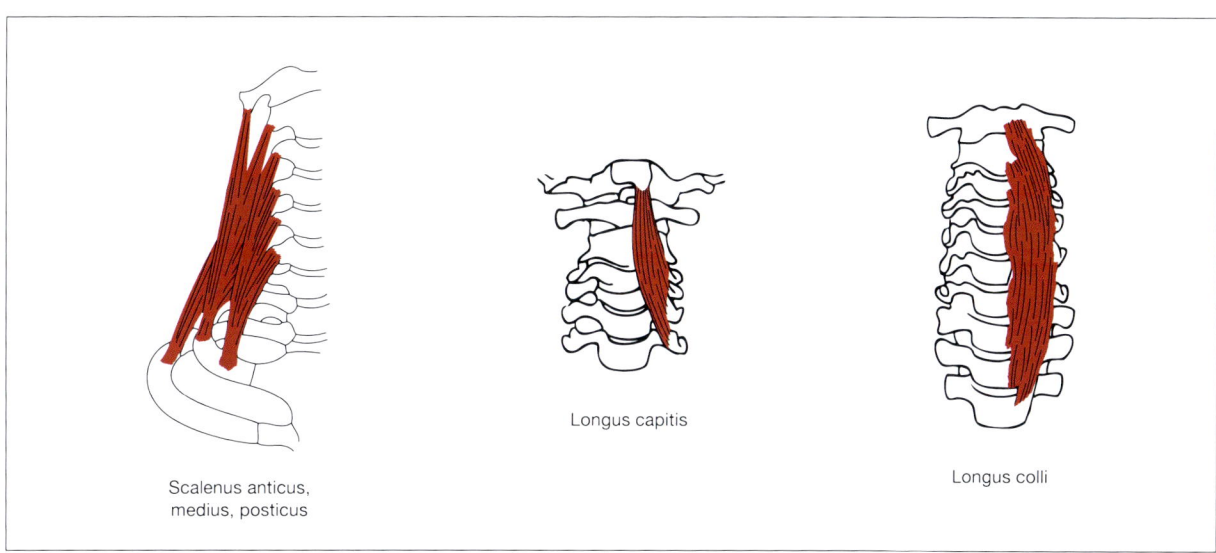

Scalenus anticus, medius, posticus

Longus capitis

Longus colli

Medial neck flexors consist of Scalenus Anticus, Scalenus Medius, and Scalenus Posticus, as well as Longus Capitus and Longus Colli.

Scalenus Anticus
Origin: anterior tubercles of the transverse processes of the C2-C6 verterbrae.
Insertion: scalene tubercle on the superior surface of rib 1, posterior to subclavian groove.
Innervation: brachial plexus C5-C8.
Action: flexion, ipsilateral lateral flexion, and contralateral rotation of the cervical spine; elevates first rib.

Scalenus Medius
Origin: posterior tubercles of transverse processes of C2-C7 vertebrae.
Insertion: superior surface of rib 1.
Innervation: brachial plexus C5-C8.
Action: flexion, ipsilateral lateral flexion and contralateral rotation of the cervical spine; elevates rib 1 on forced inspiration.

Scalenus Posticus
Origin: posterior tubercles of transverse processes of C3-C5 vertebrae.
Insertion: external border of rib 2.
Innervation: brachial plexus C7-C8.
Action: flexion, ipsilateral lateral flexion, contralateral rotation of the cervical spine.

Longus Capitus
Origin: anterior tubercles of C3-C6 cervical transverse processes.
Insertion: inferior surface of the basilar portion of the occiput.
Innervation: C1-C3 anterior rami.
Action: flexes cervical spine and head; flexes cervical vertebrae and head.

Longus Colli
Origin: the bodies of T1-T3 and C5-C7.
Insertion: bodies of C2-C4.
Innervation: C2-C6 anterior rami.
Action: flexes cervical spine and head; flexes cervical vertebrae and head.

MEDIAL NECK FLEXORS

The following applies to the medial neck flexors as a group:

CLINICAL*

- whiplash injury (origin and insertion injury)
- pain and limited range of motion with lateral flexion and rotation of the neck
- shoulder elevation problems, often contralateral to the weakness
- squamosal suture (parietal descent cranial fault)
- hyperinsulinism/insulin resistance
- sinus problems

*Courtesy of Drs. Walter Schmitt and Kerry McCord
Quintessential Applications: A(K) Clinical Protocol (QA)

Chapman's reflexes
Anterior: inferior to mid-clavicle
Posterior: C0-C2 laminae

Neurovascular point
ramus of mandible

Nutrition
vitamin B6 with niacinamide or niacin (5:1 ratio) organic iodine for sinusitis

Acupuncture meridian association
stomach

Common subluxations
upper cervicals and cranial faults

Meric TS line
rib 1 and T1

Associated point
T12, L1 (stomach)

Visceral association
sinuses

POSTURE

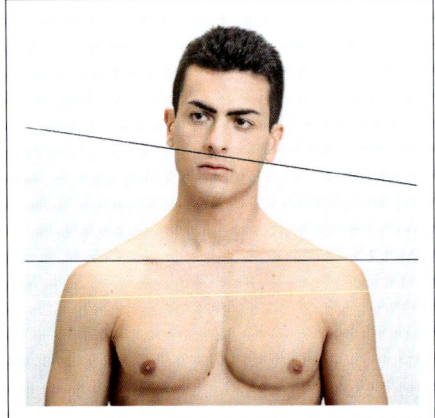

Unilateral weakness: elevation of head (occiput) on side of weakness, with slight rotation toward side of weakness.

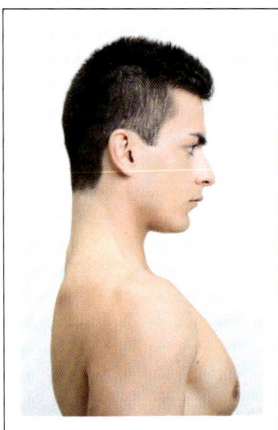

Bilateral weakness: military neck.

MEDIAL NECK FLEXORS

Test

The test is best performed supine in the following positions:

Position 1
Keeping the chin tucked, the patient lifts head off the table by maximally flexing the cervical spine then rotating the head 10 degrees away from the side being tested. The examiner places one hand under the head to catch it if it should suddenly fall back down toward the table. With the hypothenar of the other hand, contact is made on the forehead in line with the origins of the muscles, and pressure is directed toward neck extension.

Position 2
The same test is repeated with the patient's arms in 90 degrees of abduction and forearms in 90 degrees of flexion.

N.B.
Sometimes the neck flexors are only found to be weak when the arms are above head. Therefore the test should be done first with the arms at the sides. Then only if no weakness was found should the test be repeated with the arms above the head.

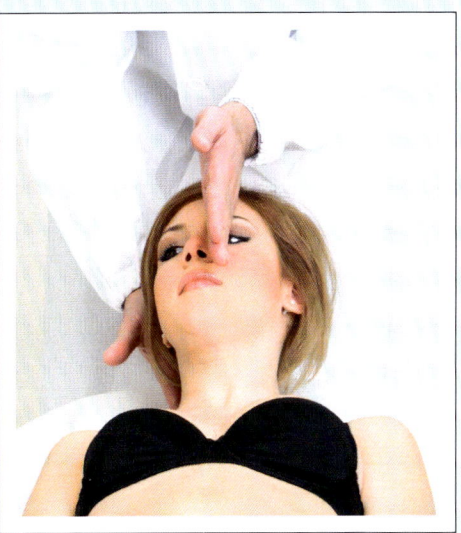

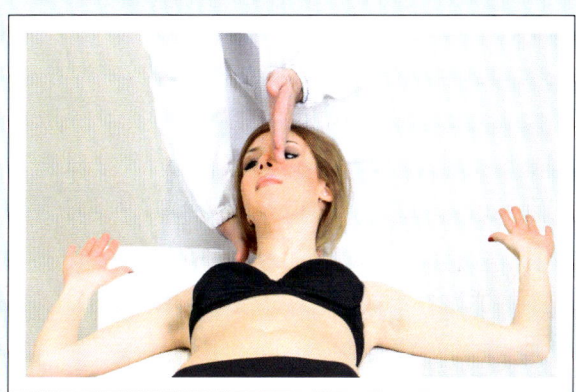

Common error

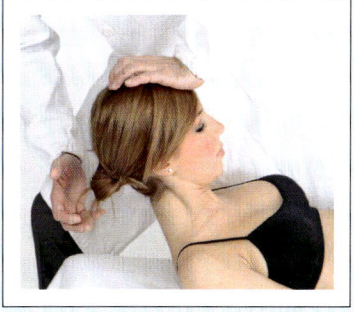

Test pressure is directed straight down toward table instead of in a cephalad vector, in line with the fibers of the muscle.

NECK EXTENSORS

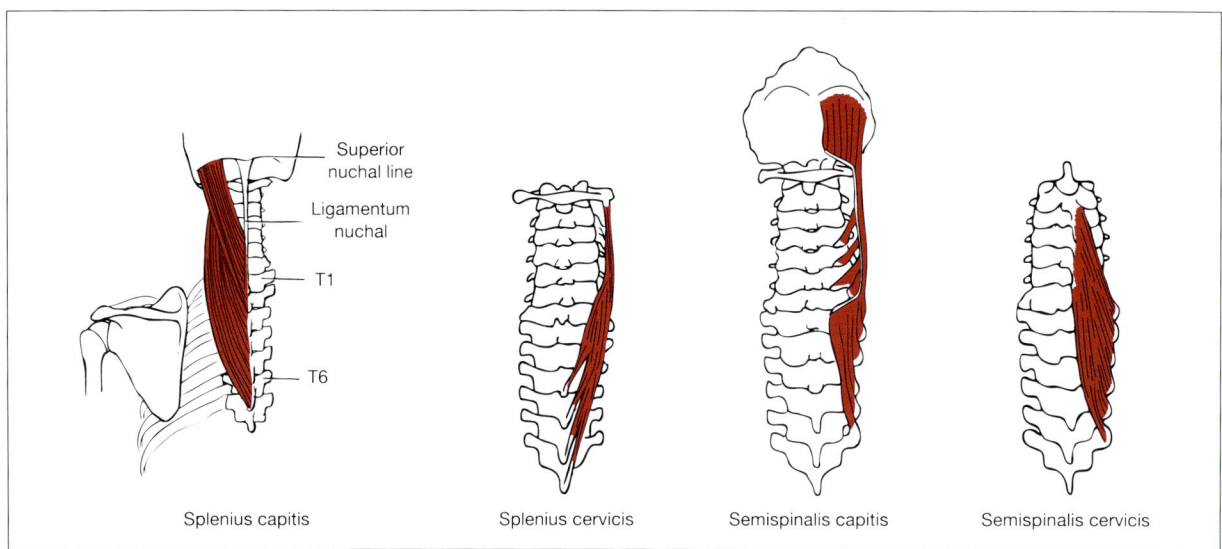

Splenius capitis   Splenius cervicis   Semispinalis capitis   Semispinalis cervicis

The neck extensors consist of the Splenius Capitis, Splenius Cervicis, Semispinalis Capitis, and Semispinalis Cervicis.

Splenius Capitis

Origin: spinous processes of C7-T3; ligamentum nuchae.

Insertion: mastoid process; lateral third of superior nuchal line.

Innervation: middle cervical spinal nerves.

Action: extension, lateral flexion, and rotation of head and neck ipsilaterally; acting bilaterally they extend the neck.

Splenius Cervicis

Origin: spinous processes of T3-T6.

Insertion: posterior transverse processes of C1-C4.

Innervation: lower cervical spinal nerves.

Action: extension, lateral flexion, and rotation of neck ipsilaterally; acting bilaterally they extend the neck.

Semispinalis Capitis

Origin: transverse processes of C7-T6; articular processes of C4-C6.

Insertion: between inferior and superior nuchal lines of the occiput.

Innervation: spinal nerves C1-C6.

Action: extension, lateral flexion, and rotation of head and neck ipsilaterally.

Semispinalis Cervicis

Origin: transverse processes of T1-T6.

Insertion: spinous processes of C2-C5.

Innervation: spinal nerves C6-C8.

Action: extension, lateral flexion, and rotation of head and neck ipsilaterally.

NECK EXTENSORS

CLINICAL*

- unilateral weakness is related to iliac fixation
- bilateral weakness is related to sacral fixation
- weak as a unit (group test) is related to lumbar fixation
- whiplash injury (origin and insertion injury)

*Courtesy of Drs. Walter Schmitt and Kerry McCord
Quintessential Applications: A(K) Clinical Protocol (QA)

Chapman's reflexes
Anterior: inferior to mid-clavicle
Posterior: C1/C2 laminae

Neurovascular point
ramus of mandible

Nutrition
vitamin B6 with niacinamide or niacin; organic iodine for sinusitis.

Meric TS line
rib 1

Acupuncture meridian association
stomach

Common subluxations
cervical spine; upper thoracic spine

Associated point
T12, L1 (stomach)

Visceral association
sinuses

POSTURE

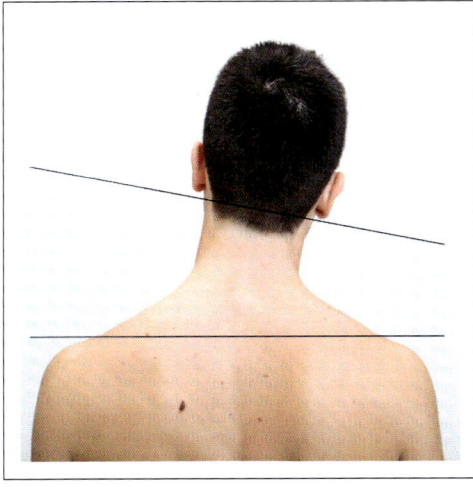

Unilateral weakness: elevation of occiput on side of weakness.

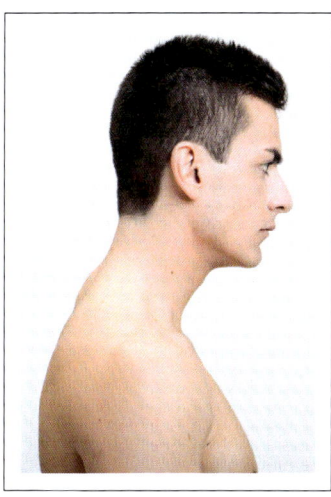

Bilateral weakness: anterior head carriage.

NECK EXTENSORS

Bilateral Neck Extensors Test group test

Position
Prone or seated.

Test
Prone patient abducts arms and flexes forearms both to 90 degrees in order to raise them off the table, then fully extends the cervical spine. Examiner contacts posterior head and directs pressure toward flexion of the cervical spine. The test pressure is cephalad, in the direction of an imaginary line with the examiner's contact hand and the patient's forehead (as opposed to straight down toward the table). When performed seated, the patient's arms are left in a relaxed position.

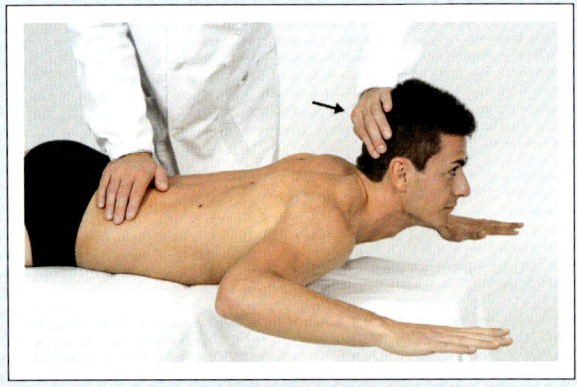
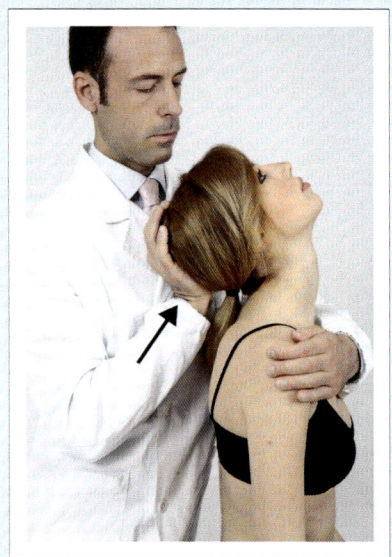

Common errors Applies to both the bilateral and unilateral tests.

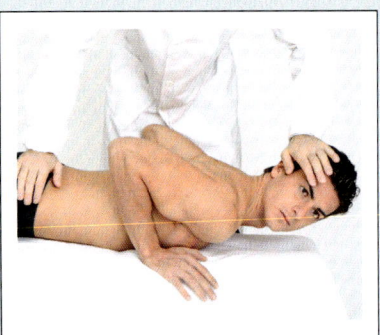

Patient is allowed to push with their hands.

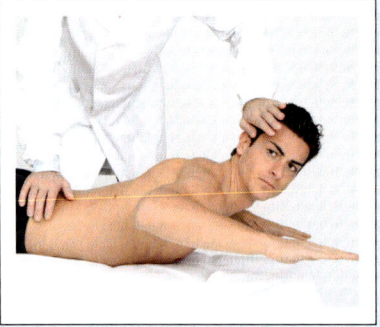

Thoracic spine is extended with chest lifted up off the table.

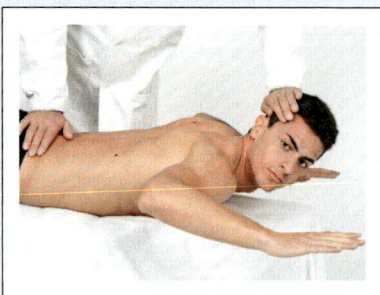

Test pressure is straight down toward table instead of cephalad.

NECK EXTENSORS

Unilateral Neck Extensors Test

Position
Prone or seated.

Test
Prone patient abducts arms and flexes forearms both to 90 degrees in order to raise them off the table, then fully extends the cervical spine and maximally rotates the head toward the side being tested. Examiner contacts the posterior, ipsilateral side of the head and directs pressure toward flexion of the cervical spine, in a cephalad vector (as opposed to straight down toward the table).

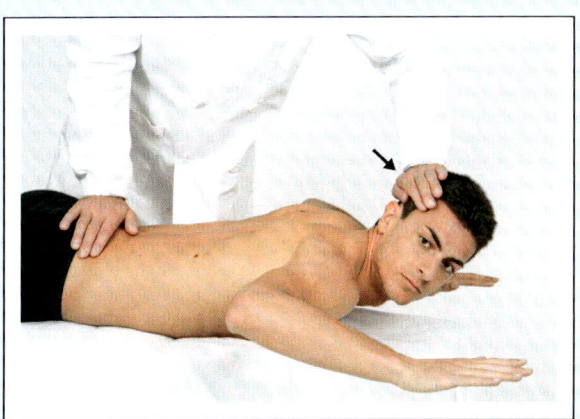
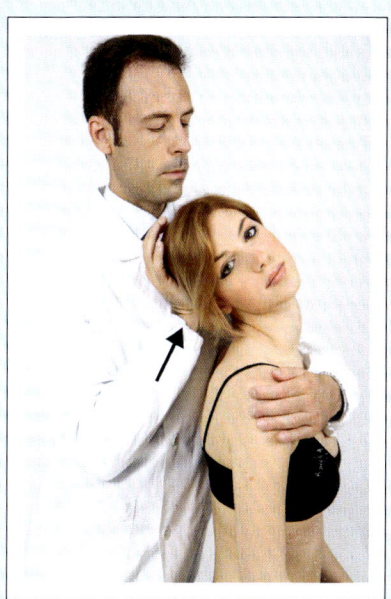

OPPONENS DIGITI MINIMI

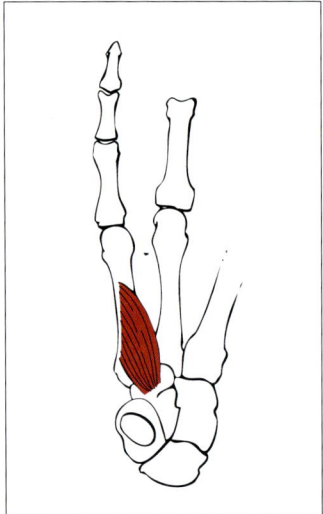

Opponens Digiti Minimi
Origin: hook of hamulate bone and flexor retinaculum.
Insertion: ulnar border of fifth metacarpal bone.
Innervation: ulnar (C7-T1).
Posterior: between PSIS and L5 spinous processes.
Action: flexes and externally rotates fifth metatarsal bone, bringing the ulnar portion of the hand toward the thumb; helps cup the hand.

CLINICAL*

- pisiform hammate syndrome (pisiform tunnel syndrome)
- difficulties with little finger

*Courtesy of Drs. W. Schmitt and K. McCord - Quintessential Applications: A(K) Clinical Protocol (QA)

Chapman's reflexes
Anterior: symphysis pubis
Posterior: ulnar border of fifth metacarpal bone

Neurovascular point
frontal bone eminences

Acupuncture meridian association
stomach

Test

Patient brings the fifth metacarpal into a position of flexion and slight external rotation to cup the palm. Examiner contacts the palmar surface of the fifth metacarpal head and directs pressure toward extension, in the direction of flattening the cupped hand.

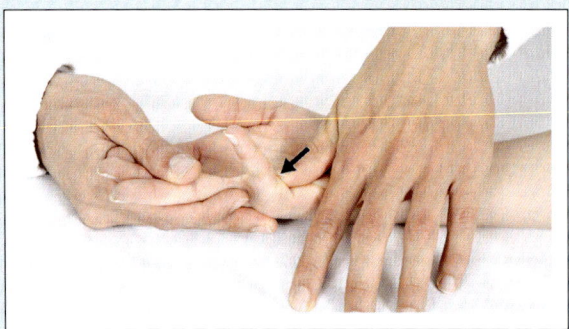
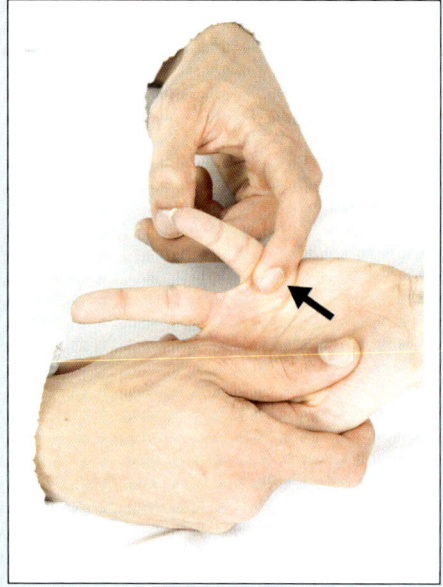

OPPONENS POLLICIS

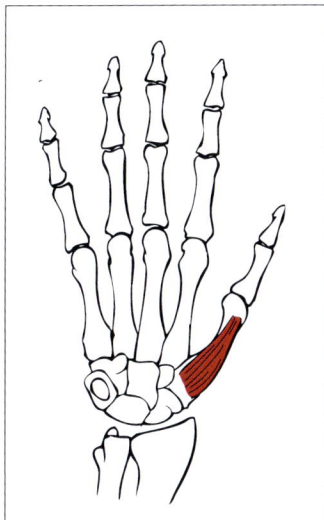

Opponens Pollicis
Origin: flexor retinaculum and tubercles of scaphoid and trapezium bones.
Insertion: radial side of entire first metacarpal bone.
Innervation: median (C6-C7).
Action: flexion and abduction of the first metacarpal bone with slight internal rotation that causes opposition of the thumb toward the center of the palm.

CLINICAL*

- carpal tunnel syndrome
- difficulty holding objects
- difficulty opening a jar

*Courtesy of Drs. W. Schmitt and K. McCord - Quintessential Applications: A(K) Clinical Protocol (QA)

Chapman's reflexes
Anterior: symphysis pubis
Posterior: between PSIS and L5 spinous process

Visceral association
stomach

Acupuncture meridian association
stomach

Test

Keeping the first metacarpophalangeal articulation in extension, patient flexes, adducts, and slightly internally rotates first metacarpal. Examiner uses one hand to stabilize either over the hypothenar eminence or over the non-tested digits, while using a finger of the other hand to direct pressure at the distal end of the first metacarpal toward extension, abduction, and external rotation.

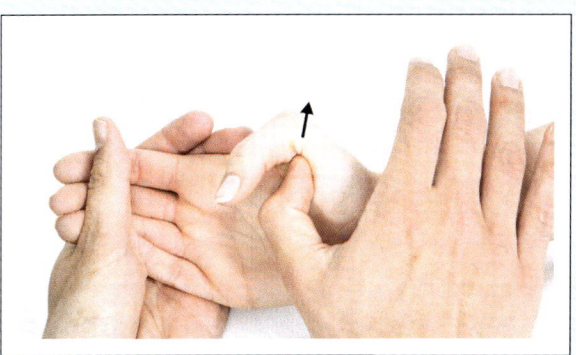

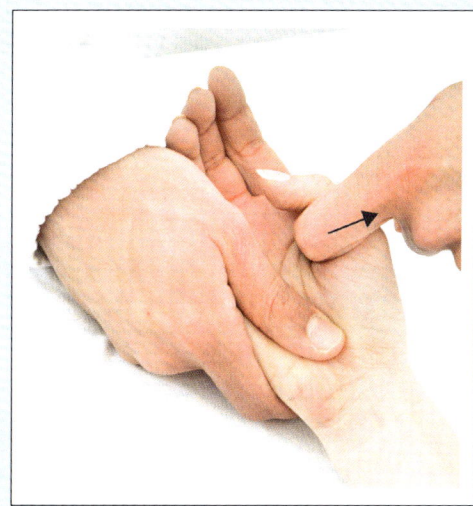

OPPONENS POLLICIS

Test for Opponens Pollicis and Opponens Digiti Minimi Together

Test
Patient brings the fifth metacarpal into a position of flexion and slight external rotation to cup the palm. Simultaneously, the first metacarpal is brought into flexion, adduction, and slight internal rotation, keeping the metacarpophalangeal articulation, as well as the non-tested digits in extension. The tips of the first and fifth digit will be touching in the starting position of the test. Examiner contacts the metacarpal shafts of the first and fifth digits, and directs pressure to separate the shafts.

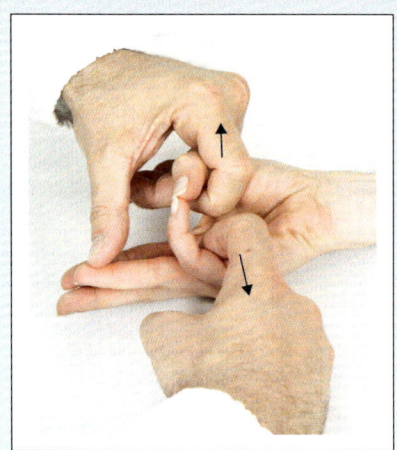

Common errors

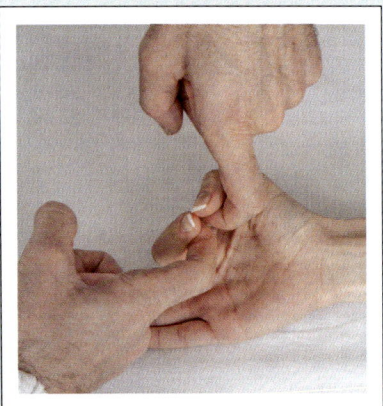 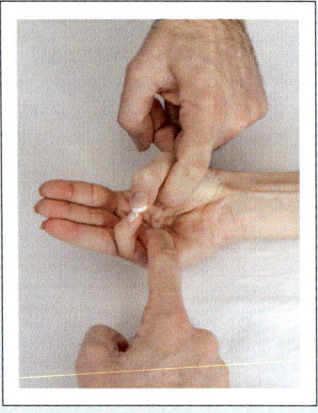

Contact is made at the distal digits (as in the O-ring test).

Patient is allowed to flex the non-tested fingers.

PECTORALIS MAJOR CLAVICULAR

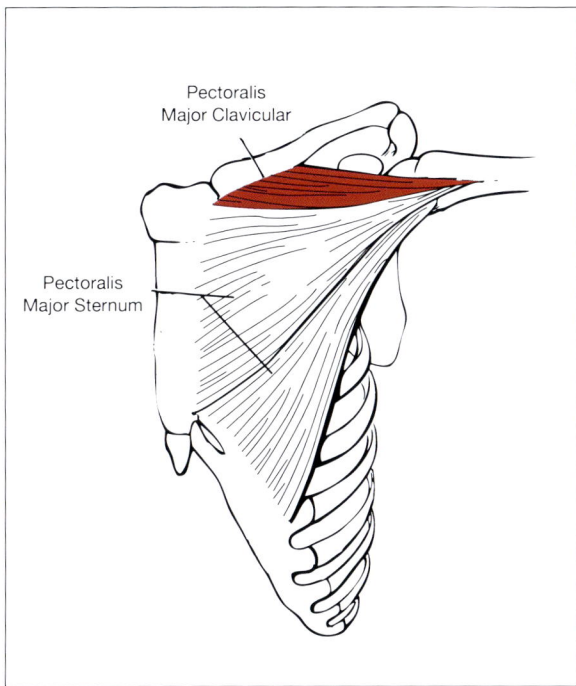

Pectoralis Major Clavicular
Origin: anterior surface of medial half of clavicle.
Insertion: lateral lip of the intertubercular groove of the humerus.
Innervation: lateral pectoral (C5-C7).
Action: flexes and horizontally adducts humerus toward the opposite shoulder; in some people it internally rotates humerus.

Chapman's reflexes
Anterior: left 5th and 6th intercostal spaces
Posterior: left T5, T6, and T7

Neurovascular point
frontal bone eminences

Nutrition
betaine hydrochloride; stomach substance with B-12; "B" and "G"

Acupuncture meridian association
stomach

Common subluxations
C5, C6, and C7

Meric TS line
T5

Associated point
T12, L1 (stomach)

Visceral association
stomach

CLINICAL*

- throwing problems
- emotional stress
- B-vitamin deficiency symptoms (GERD, H-pylori, etc.)
- bilateral weakness associated with allergies, HCl need, temporal bulge cranial fault

*Courtesy of Drs. Walter Schmitt and Kerry McCord
Quintessential Applications: A(K) Clinical Protocol (QA)

PECTORALIS MAJOR CLAVICULAR

POSTURE

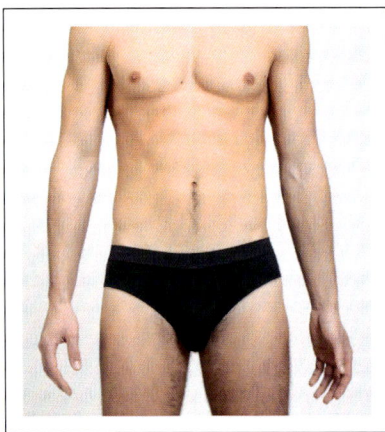

Arm, forearm and hand hang in external rotation. The palm will either face forward or in less extreme cases, the hand will rotate externally from the frontal plane.

Test

Position
Supine, seated, or standing.

Test
Patient extends forearm, locking it at the elbow, flexes humerus to 90 degrees, and internally rotates humerus so that thumb faces in the direction of the feet (the degree of internal rotation will depend upon the anatomical formation of the individual patient's shoulder). Examiner contacts the lateral surface of the distal forearm and uses it as a lever to direct pressure toward abduction and slight extension of the humerus.

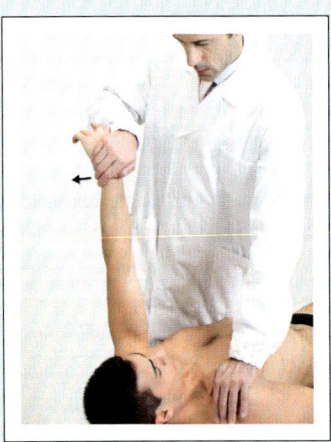
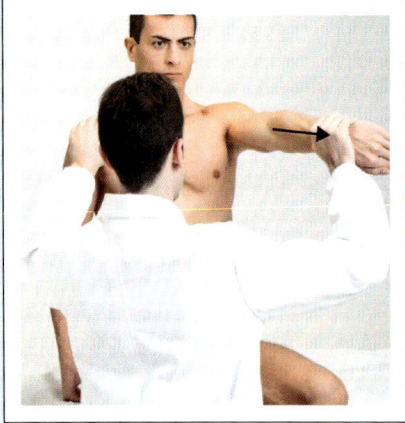

PECTORALIS MAJOR CLAVICULAR

Common errors

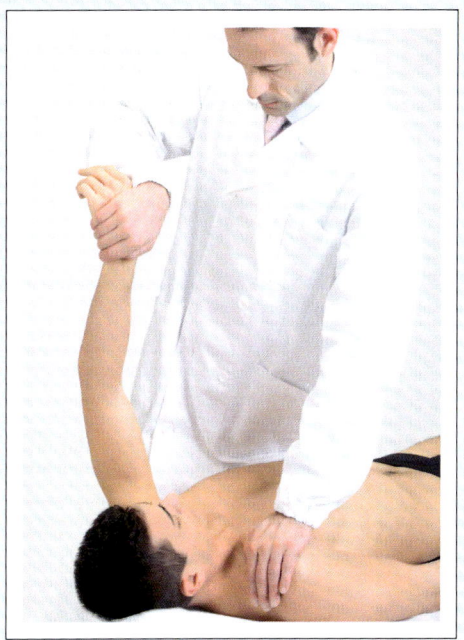

Elbow is allowed to bend.

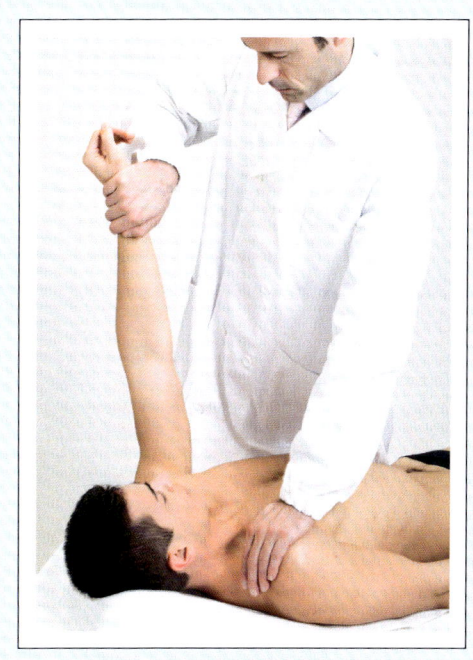

Arm is allowed to laterally rotate.

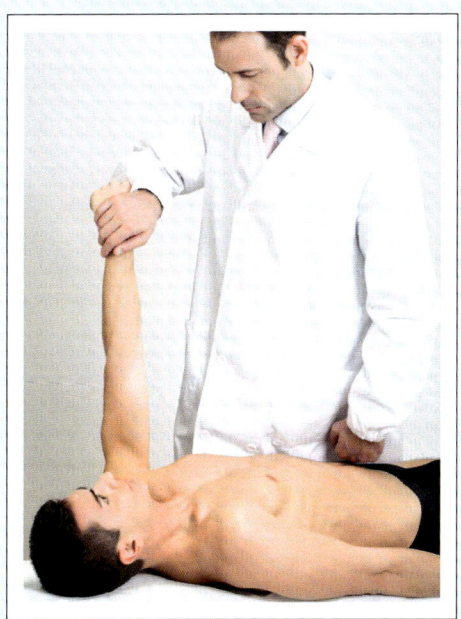

No stabilization.

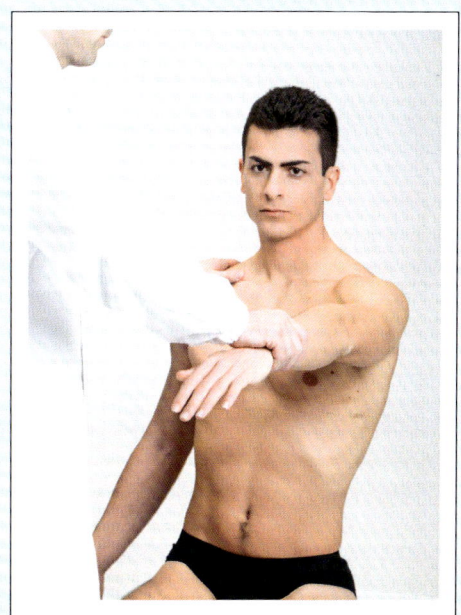

Confused with "arm pull down test".

PECTORALIS MAJOR STERNUM

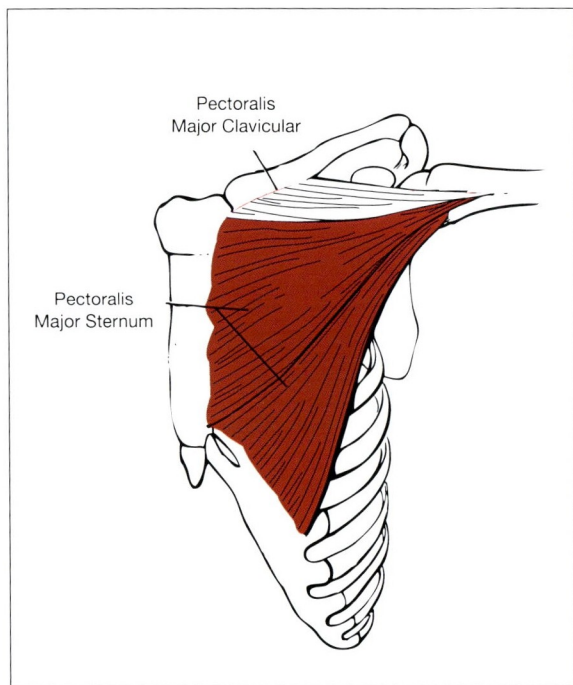

Pectoralis Major Sternum
Origin: anterior surface of sternum; superior 6 costal cartilages; aponeurosis of external abdominal oblique muscle.
Insertion: lateral lip of the intertubercular groove of the humerus.
Innervation: medial and lateral pectoral (C6-T1).
Action: adducts humerus toward opposite iliac crest; the sternal fibers extend shoulder joint from a flexed position; stabilizes shoulder anteriorly.

Chapman's reflexes
Anterior: right 5th and 6th intercostal spaces
Posterior: right T5 and T6

Neurovascular point
one and a half inches up from prominent bulges on frontal bones, one and a half inches from midline

Nutrition
vitamin A; bile salts; liver tissue; any liver detoxification substances

Acupuncture meridian association
liver

Common subluxations
C7-T1

Meric TS line
T8

Associated point
T9 and T10 (liver)

Visceral association
liver

CLINICAL*

- Rhomboid tightness ipsilaterally
- throwing problems
- vitamin A symptoms: night blindness, other visual disturbances
- fat metabolism (increased cholesterol and/or triglycerides)
- liver associated problems: biliary; detoxification problems

*Courtesy of Drs. Walter Schmitt and Kerry McCord
Quintessential Applications: A(K) Clinical Protocol (QA)

PECTORALIS MAJOR STERNUM

POSTURE

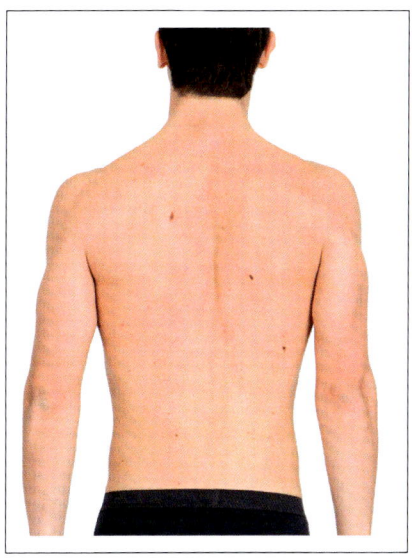

Visibly tight ipsilateral rhomboid (ipsilateral scapula elevated).

Test

Position
Supine.

Test
Patient extends forearm, locking it at the elbow, flexes (to 90 degrees) and internally rotates humerus so that thumb points in the direction of the feet (the degree of internal rotation will depend upon the anatomical formation of the individual patient's shoulder). Examiner stabilizes over the contralateral ASIS with one hand, while the other hand contacts the lateral surface of the distal forearm and uses it as a lever to direct pressure toward abduction and increased flexion of the humerus.

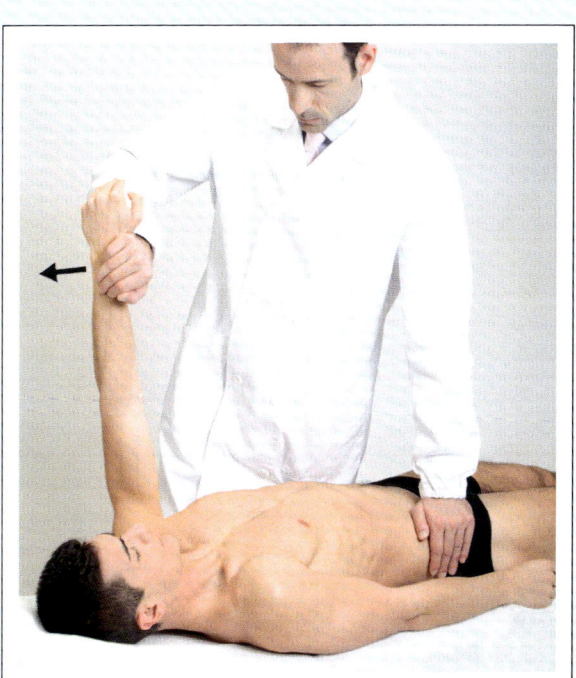

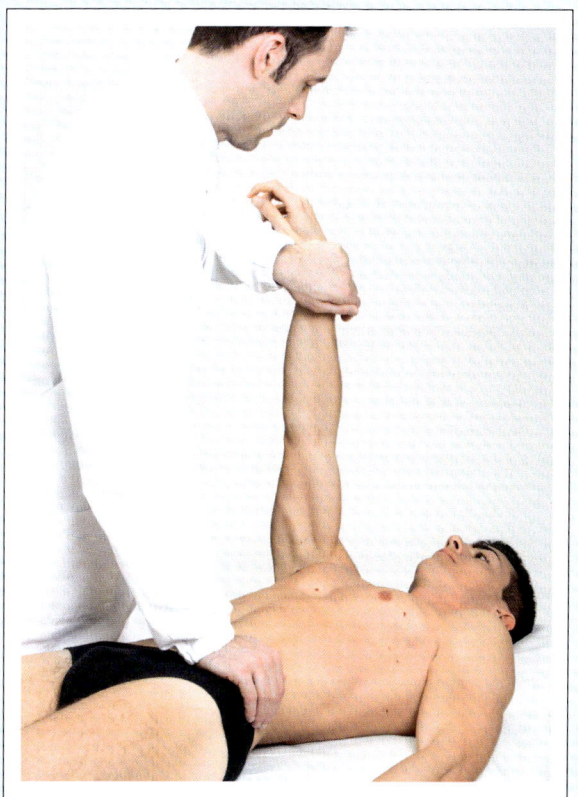

PECTORALIS MAJOR STERNUM

Common errors

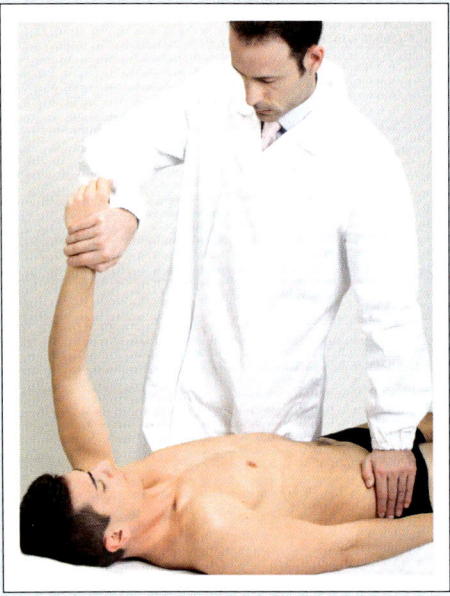

Elbow is allowed to bend.

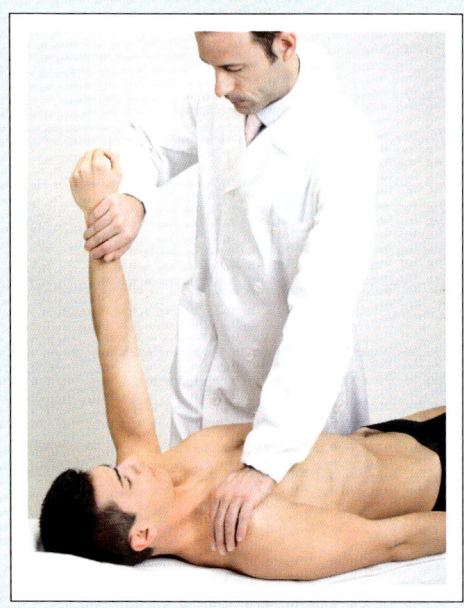

Stabilization at the opposite shoulder (confused with pectoralis major clavicular).

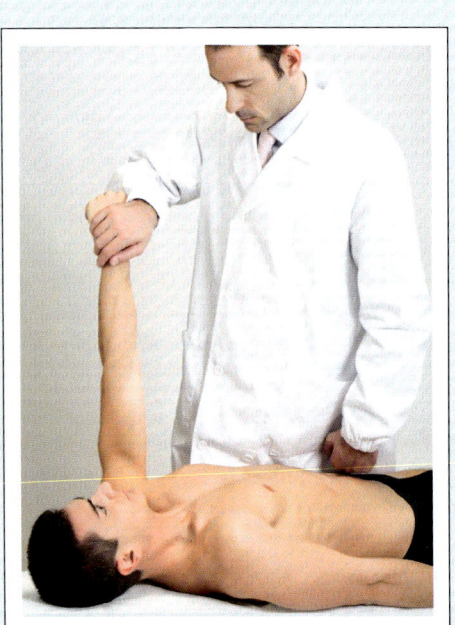

No stabilization.

PECTORALIS MINOR

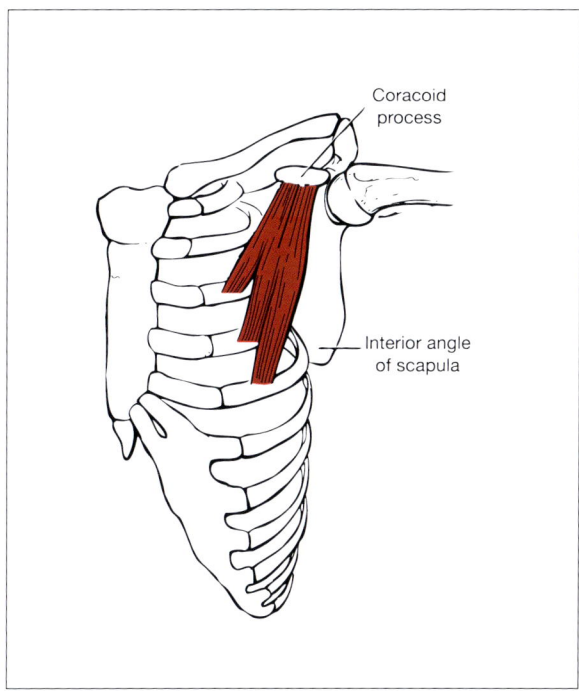

Pectoralis Minor

Origin: ribs 3 to 5 near their costal cartilages.

Insertion: coracoid process of scapula.

Innervation: medial pectoral (C7-T1).

Action: stabilizes scapula by drawing it anteriorly, medially, and inferiorly against thoracic wall.

CLINICAL*

- shoulder injury from punching motions
- chemical hypersensitivities
- heavy metal toxicity
- AK retrograde lymph problems

*Courtesy of Drs. Walter Schmitt and Kerry McCord
Quintessential Applications: A(K) Clinical Protocol (QA)

Chapman's reflexes
Anterior 1: lower half of sternum
Anterior 2: 2nd, 3rd, 4th, and 5th intercostal spaces

Nutrition
molybdenum; parotid tissue;
iron;
vitamin F (essential fatty acids);
any anti-heavy metal substance

Acupuncture meridian association
large intestine

Common subluxations
C6-T1

Visceral association
parotid gland/immune system

PECTORALIS MINOR

Test 1

Position
Supine.

Test
Patient lifts shoulder off the table by drawing coracoid process anteriorly, medially, and inferiorly. Examiner contacts the anterior surface of the shoulder and directs pressure posteriorly in a vector toward elongation of the pectoralis minor muscle fibers.

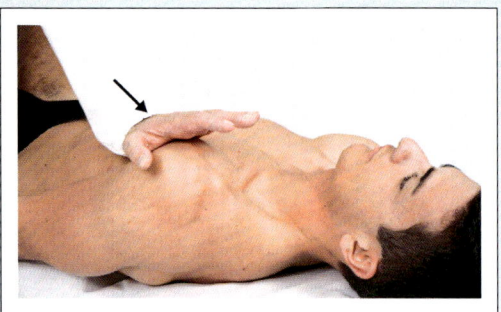

Test 2 Alternate Test

Position
Supine.

Test
Patient fully extends arm, locking it at the elbow, then slightly flexes and adducts humerus so that the medial forearm lies over umbilicus, and the hypothenar over the contralateral ASIS. In this position the thumb is pointing toward the ceiling. Examiner contacts the medial, distal forearm and uses it as a lever, directing pressure straight upward toward the ceiling to impart pressure toward flexion and abduction of the humerus.

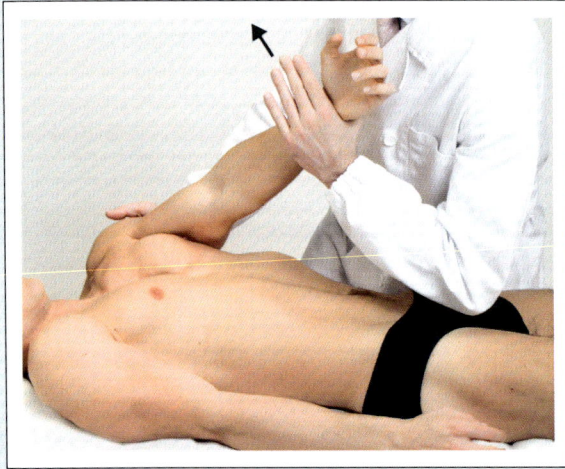
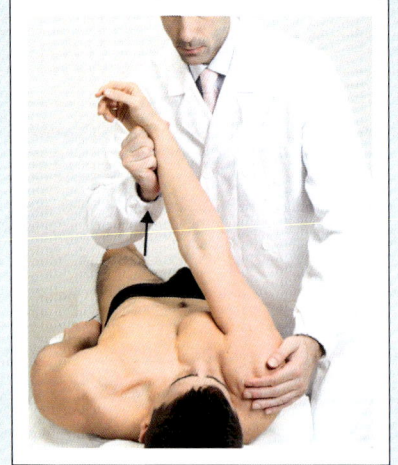

PERONEUS BREVIS

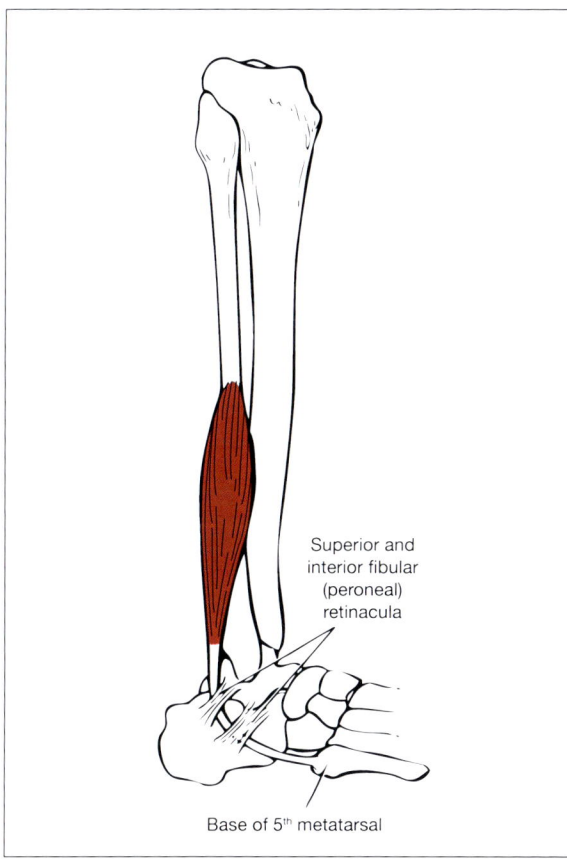

Superior and interior fibular (peroneal) retinacula

Base of 5th metatarsal

Peroneus Brevis
Origin: inferior two-thirds of lateral surface of fibula and adjacent intermuscular septum.

Insertion: lateral surface of proximal end of fifth metatarsal.

Innervation: peroneal L4-S1.

Action: plantarflexes and everts foot; lends lateral stability to the ankle.

Chapman's reflexes
Anterior: inferior pubic bone
Posterior: L5/PSIS

Neurovascular point
frontal bone eminences

Nutrition
vitamin B-complex; calcium

Acupuncture meridian association
bladder

Common subluxations
L4, L5, and S1

Associated point
S1 (bladder)

Visceral association
urinary bladder

CLINICAL*

- origin and insertion injuries in inversion ankle sprain (allows recurrent injuries)
- fifth metatarsal and lateral foot symptoms
- bladder

*Courtesy of Drs. Walter Schmitt and Kerry McCord
Quintessential Applications: A(K) Clinical Protocol (QA)

PERONEUS BREVIS

Test

Position
Supine or seated.

Test
With teeth lightly clenched and toes in flexion, patient maximally plantarflexes and everts foot. Examiner uses one hand to stabilize just proximal to the medial malleolus, while the other hand contacts the lateral surface of the foot and directs pressure toward inversion and dorsiflexion.

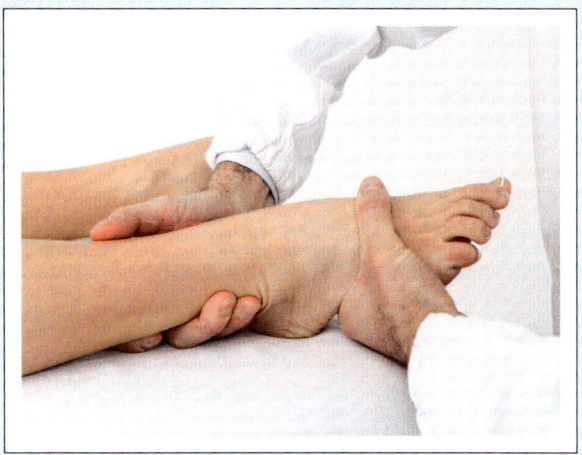

Common error

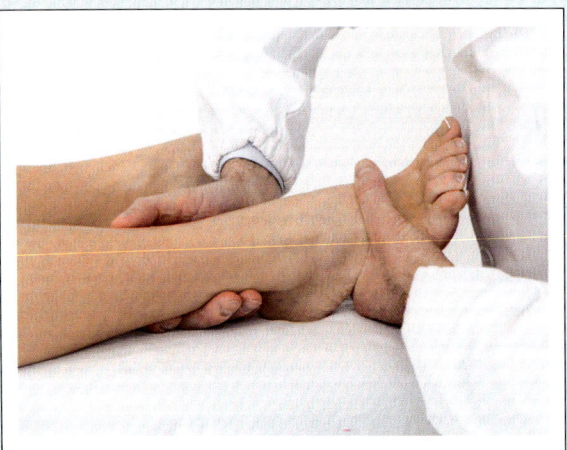

Toes allowed to dorsiflex.

PERONEUS LONGUS

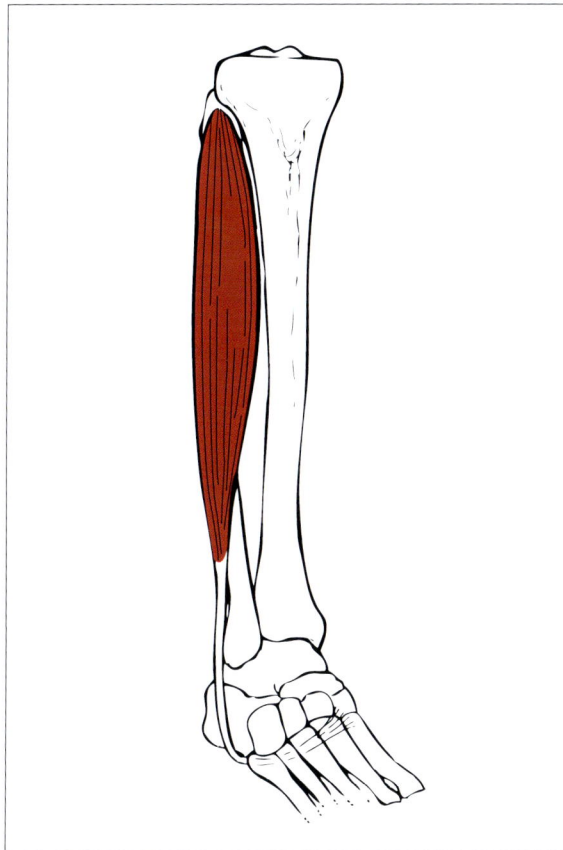

Peroneus Longus
Origin: lateral condyle of tibia; head and proximal two-thirds of lateral surface of fibula; intermuscular septa and adjacent fascia.

Insertion: proximal end of first metatarsal and medial cuneiform on their lateral portions.

Innervation: peroneal L4-S1.

Action: plantarflexes and everts foot; lends lateral stability to the ankle.

Chapman's reflexes
Anterior: inferior pubic bone
Posterior: L5/PSIS

Neurovascular point
frontal bone eminences

Nutrition
vitamin B-complex; calcium

Acupuncture meridian association
bladder

Common subluxations
L4, L5, and S1

Associated point
S1 (bladder)

Visceral association
urinary bladder

CLINICAL*

- origin and insertion injuries in inversion ankle sprain (allows recurrent injuries)
- subluxations: navicular, first cuneiform, first metatarsal
- fibular pain sometimes described as lateral knee pain
- bladder

*Courtesy of Drs. Walter Schmitt and Kerry McCord Quintessential Applications: A(K) Clinical Protocol (QA)

PERONEUS LONGUS

Test

Position
Supine.

Test
With teeth lightly clenched and the toes kept in neutral position, patient partly plantarflexes and maximally everts the foot. Examiner uses both hands to clasp around the arch of the foot then directs pressure toward inversion and dorsiflexion. The vector of test pressure is a rolling motion against the pull of the peroneus longus tendon (as opposed to a straight inversion vector).

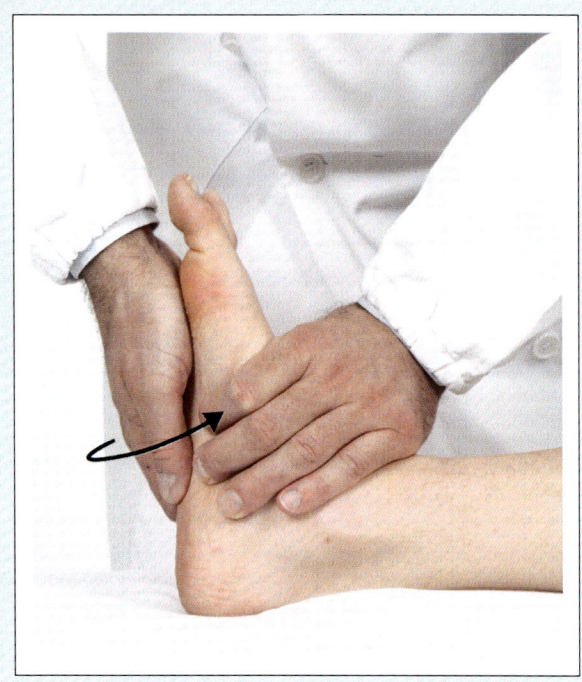

Common error

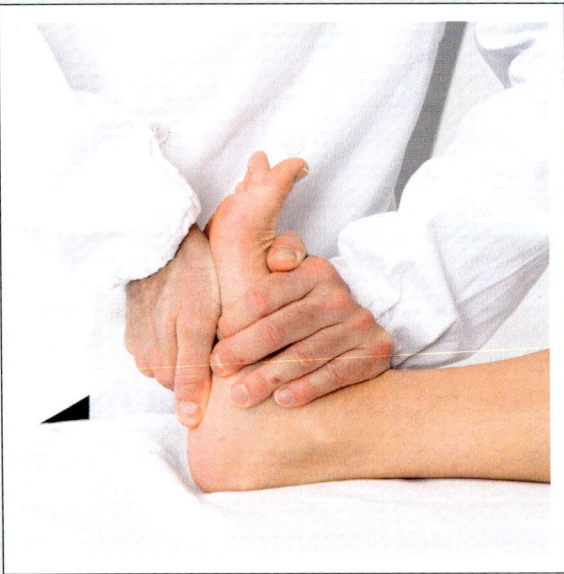

Toes allowed to dorsiflex.

PERONEUS TERTIUS

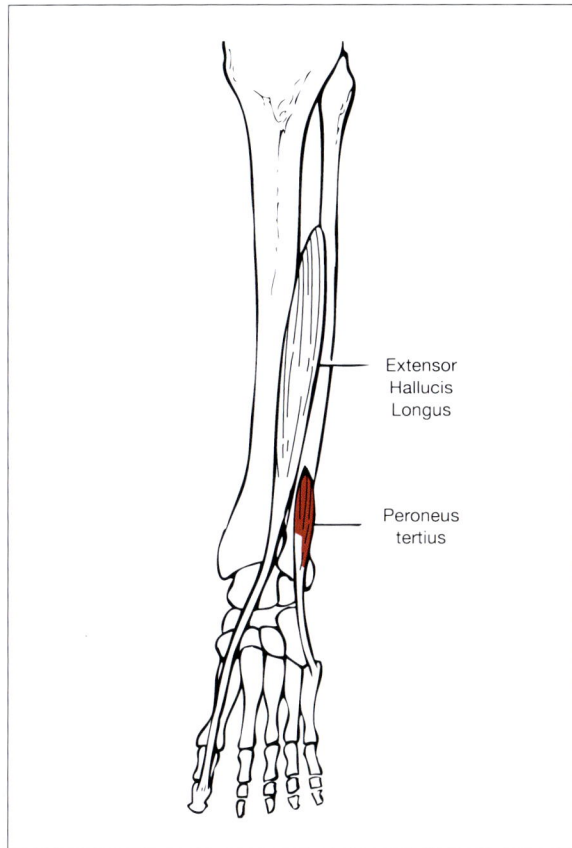

Peroneus Tertius
Origin: lower third of the anterior surface of the fibula and adjacent intermuscular septum.

Insertion: dorsal surface of the proximal end of the fifth metatarsal.

Innervation: peroneal (L4-S1).

Action: dorsiflexes and everts foot.

Chapman's reflexes
Anterior: inferior pubic bone
Posterior: L5/PSIS

Neurovascular point
frontal bone eminences

Nutrition
vitamin B-complex; calcium

Acupuncture meridian association
bladder

Common subluxations
L4, L5, and S1

Associated point
S1 (bladder)

Visceral association
urinary bladder

CLINICAL*

- origin and insertion injuries in inversion ankle sprain (allows recurrent injuries)
- fifth metatarsal and lateral foot symptoms
- cuboid and third cuneiform subluxations
- bladder

*Courtesy of Drs. Walter Schmitt and Kerry McCord
Quintessential Applications: A(K) Clinical Protocol (QA)

PERONEUS TERTIUS

POSTURE

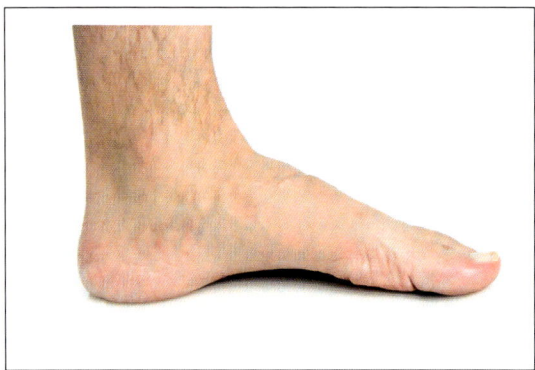

Pes cavus; supination.

Common error

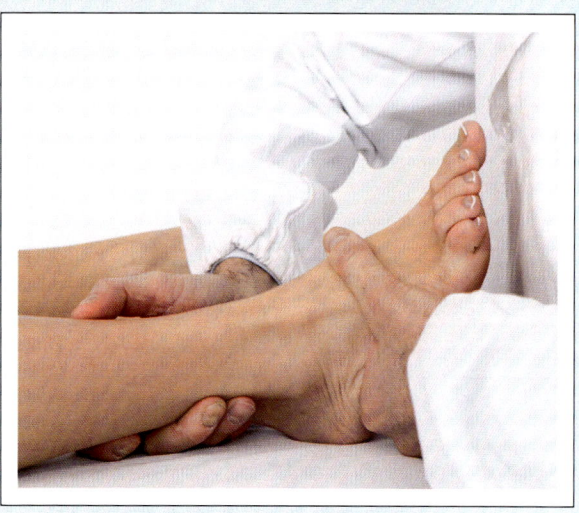

Toes are allowed to dorsiflex.

Test

Position
Supine or seated.

Test
With teeth lightly clenched and the toes kept in flexion, patient dorsiflexes and everts foot. Examiner uses one hand to stabilize over medial malleolus, while the other hand contacts the lateral surface of the dorsum of the foot to direct pressure toward plantarflexion and inversion.

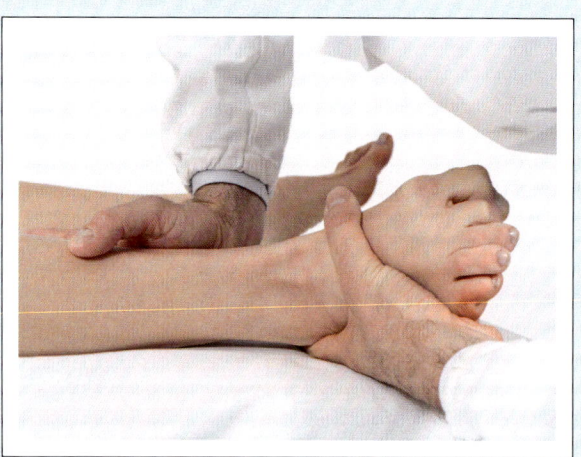

PIRIFORMIS

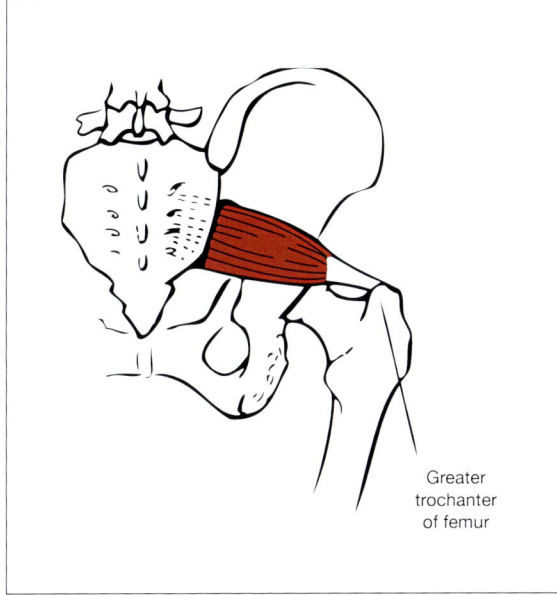

Greater trochanter of femur

Piriformis
Origin: anterior surface of sacrum - between and lateral to - anterior sacral foramen; capsule of sacroilliac articulation; margin of greater sciatic foramen; sacrotuberous ligament.
Insertion: superior border of greater trochanter of femur.
Innervation: sacral plexus (L5-S2).
Action: external rotation of femur; abducts flexed femur.

Chapman's reflexes
Anterior: upper pubic bone
Posterior: L5/PSIS

Neurovascular point
parietal eminence

Nutrition
vitamin E; vitamin A; female or male organ substance

Acupuncture meridian association
circulation sex

Common subluxations
L5 and sacrum

Meric TS line
L5

Associated point
T4 and T5 (circulation sex)

Visceral association
T4 and T5 (circulation sex)

CLINICAL*

- greater trochanter pain
- weak on the side of sciatica "drops down" on sciatic nerve
- greater foot turn in on inhibited side
- sacrum subluxation and subsequent neck pain

*Courtesy of Drs. Walter Schmitt and Kerry McCord
Quintessential Applications: A(K) Clinical Protocol (QA)

PIRIFORMIS

POSTURE

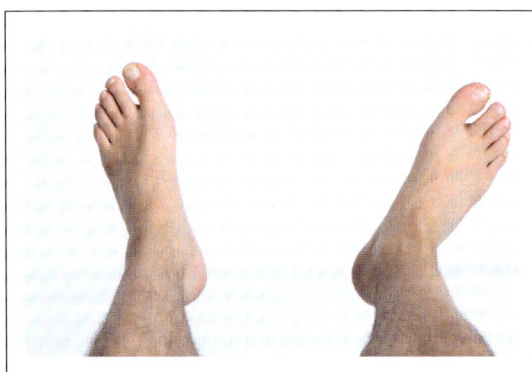

Foot rotated outward on side contralateral to weakness - best seen supine.

Test

Position
Best tested prone, but can be performed supine or seated.

Test
Prone patient bends leg to 90 degrees and externally rotates femur (the degree of external rotation may be varied).
Examiner stands on the side being tested and uses one hand to stabilize over the contralateral, posterior ilium while the other hand contacts the medial, distal leg and uses it as a lever to affect pressure toward internal rotation of the femur by pulling away from the midline.

N.B. If tested supine, the starting position is the same but with an added 20 degrees of femur abduction.

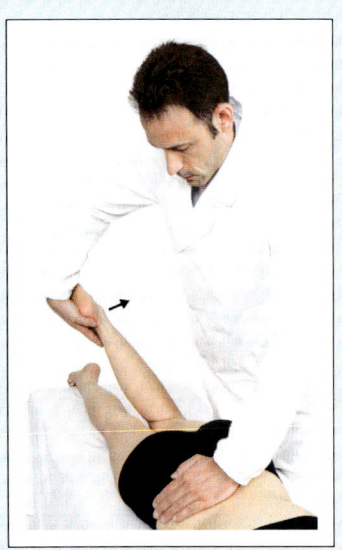
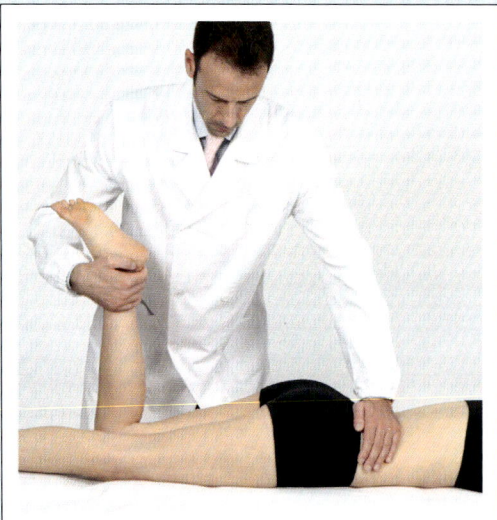
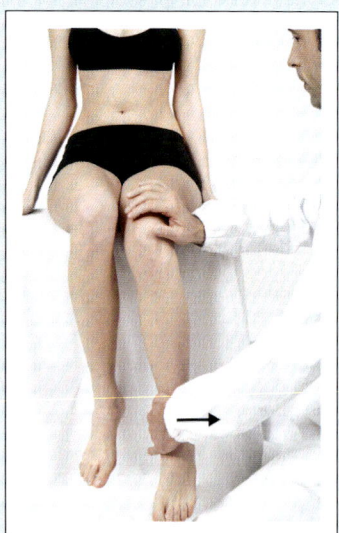

PIRIFORMIS

Common errors

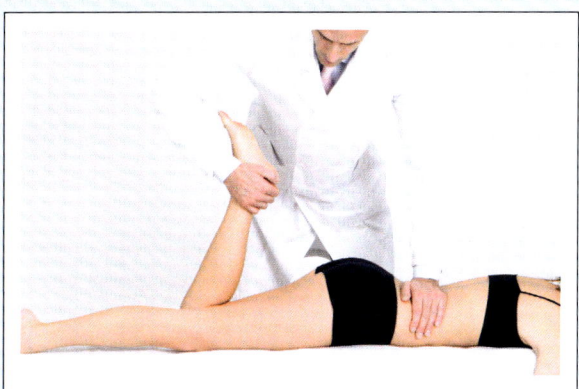

Leg is not maintained at 90 degrees (too much flexion).

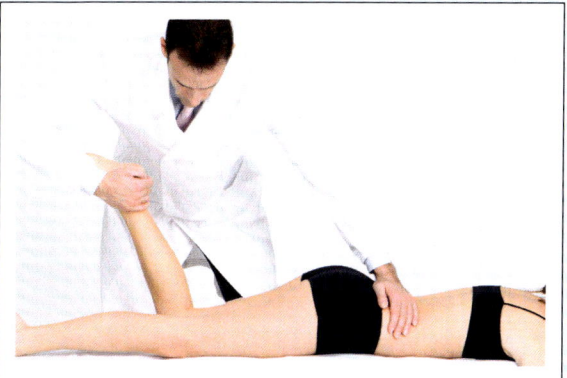

Leg is not maintained at 90 degrees (too much extension).

POPLITEUS

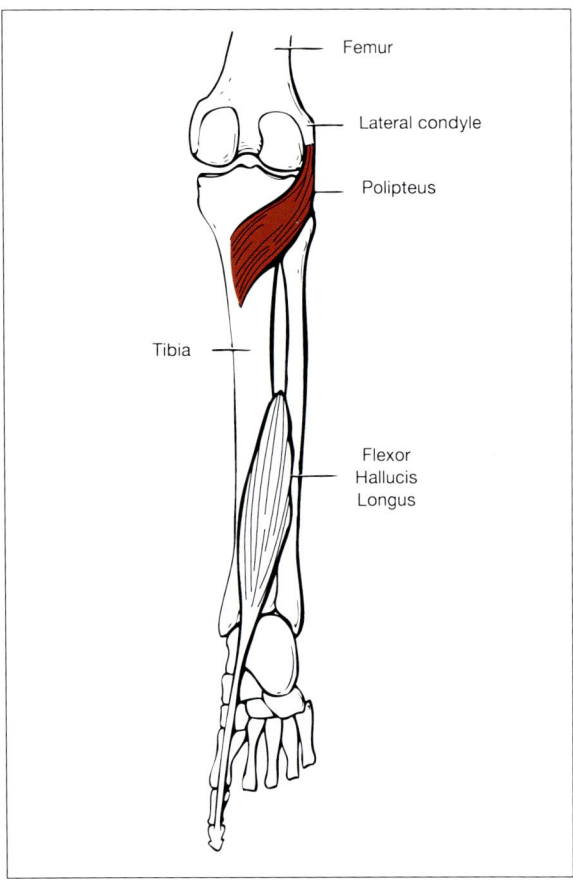

Popliteus

Origin: lateral surface of lateral condyle of femur; posterior horn of lateral meniscus; fibular head.

Insertion: posterior surface of tibia superior to soleal line.

Innervation: tibial (L4-S1).

Action: internally rotates tibia on the femur or externally rotates femur on the tibia, depending on which one is fixed; withdraws the meniscus during flexion of the leg; provides rotatory stability to the femur on the tibia; brings the knee out of the "screw home" position of full extension; gives posterior stability to the knee.

CLINICAL*

- difficulty going down stairs
- any knee problems
- gallbladder

*Courtesy of Drs. Walter Schmitt and Kerry McCord
Quintessential Applications: A(K) Clinical Protocol (QA)

Chapman's reflexes
Anterior: right 4th and 5th intercostal space from the sternum to the mid-mamillary line
Posterior: T4, T5, T6

Neurovascular point
medial aspect of the knee at the meniscus

Nutrition
bile salts; vitamin A

Acupuncture meridian association
gall bladder

Common subluxations
L4, L5 and S1

Meric TS line
T4

Associated point
T10 and T11 (gall bladder)

Visceral association
gallbladder

POPLITEUS

POSTURE

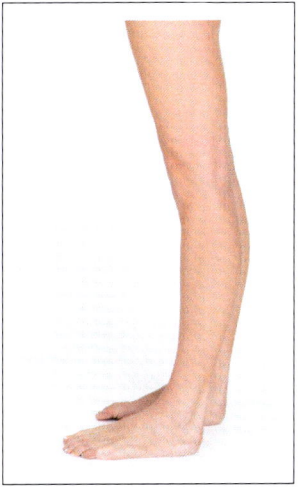

Stands with knee in hyperextension.

Test

Position
Seated, supine, or prone.

Test
In prone position, patient lightly clenches teeth and flexes leg to 90 degrees. Examiner places one hand on the distal, medial surface of the foot and the other hand around the posterior calcaneus. The foot is used as a lever to impart lateral rotational force of the tibia on the femur. This is done by directing pressure through both hands in a twisting motion toward lateral rotation of the foot. It is essential to observe for rotation at the tibial tubercle which would indicate a positive test.

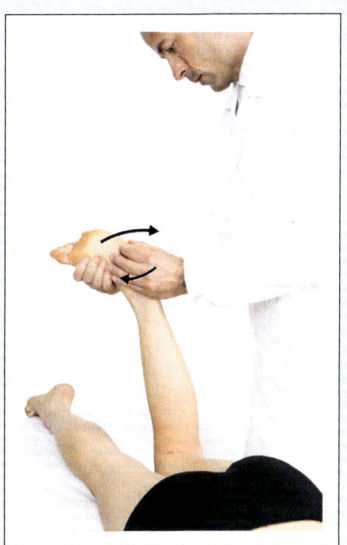
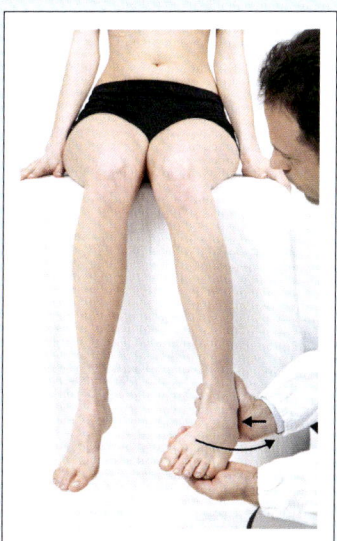

Common error

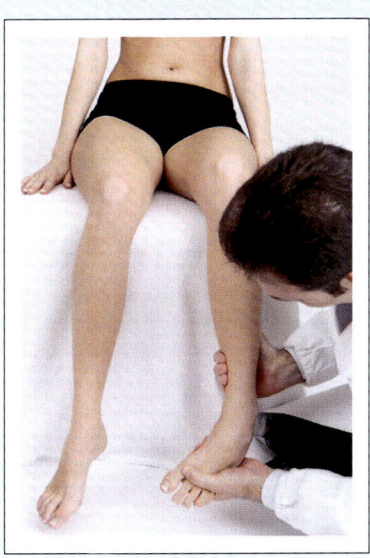

Examiner fails to observe for rotation at the tibial tubercle and instead concludes that the test is positive on the basis of lateral foot rotation.

POSTERIOR TIBIALIS

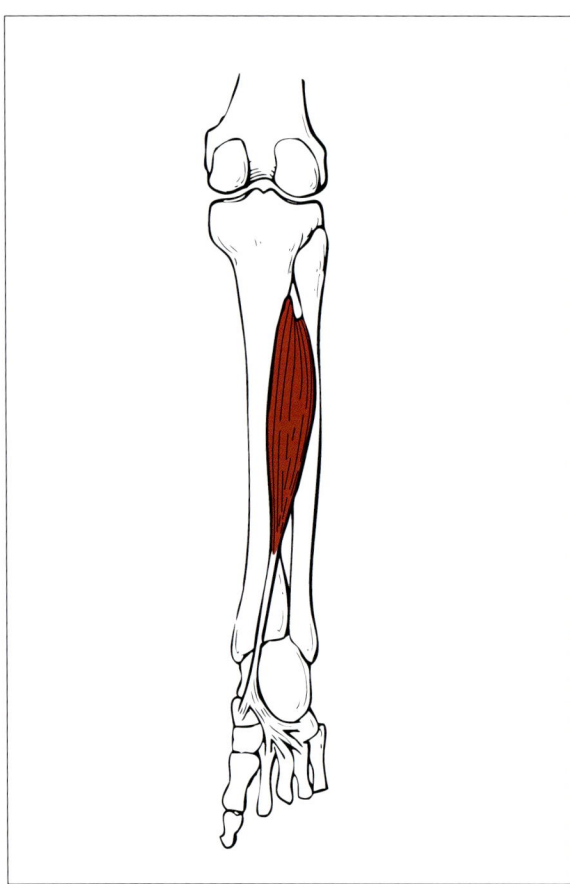

Posterior Tibialis
Origin: lateral surface of posterior tibia; medial two-thirds of posterior fibula; interosseous membrane.
Insertion: tuberosity of navicular; plantar surface of all cuneiforms bones; cuboid bone; sustentaculum tali, and plantar surfaces of the bases of second, third, fourth metatarsal bones.
Innervation: tibial (L4-S1).
Action: plantar flexes and inverts foot (maintains arch and pulls it superiorly during step); medial ankle stabilizer.

Chapman's reflexes
Anterior: 1 inch lateral and 2 inches superior to umbillicus
Posterior: T11 and T12

Neurovascular point
lambda

Nutrition
adrenal substance; vitamin C; pantothenic acid; niacinamide; wheat germ oil; DHEA; adaptogens

Acupuncture meridian association
circulation sex (pericardium)

Common subluxations
L4-S2

Meric TS line
T9

Associated point
T4 and T5 (circulation sex)

Visceral association
adrenals

POSTURE

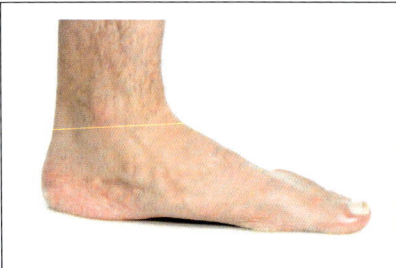

Pes planus "flat feet" and/or foot pronation.

POSTERIOR TIBIALIS

CLINICAL*

- most common foot and ankle weakness
- foot pronation and/or flat feet
- essential to foot and ankle stability
- recurrent foot subluxations
- symptoms of tired feet
- no "spring in the step"
- plantar fasciitis
- posterior shin splints
- wobbly ankle
- hammer toes
- tarsal tunnel syndrome
- adrenals

*Courtesy of Drs. Walter Schmitt and Kerry McCord
Quintessential Applications: A(K) Clinical Protocol (QA)

Test

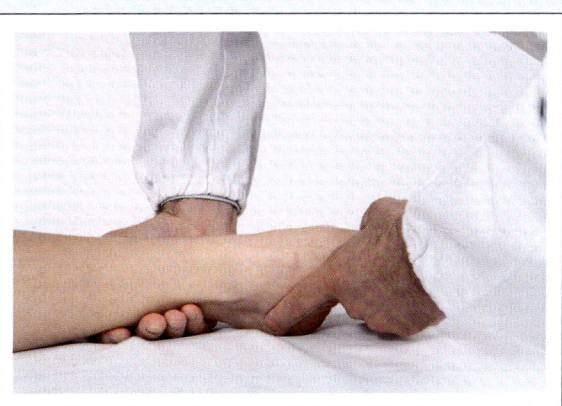

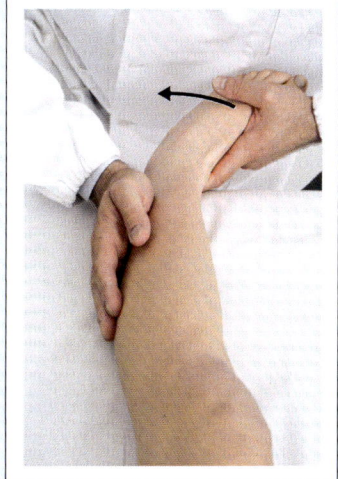

Position
Supine or seated.

Test
Keeping the toes in flexion, patient maximally plantarflexes then inverts foot. Examiner uses one hand to stabilize over the lateral malleolus, while the other hand contacts the medial surface of the foot and directs pressure toward eversion and dorsiflexion in a rolling type movement (as opposed to a straight lateral vector).

Common error

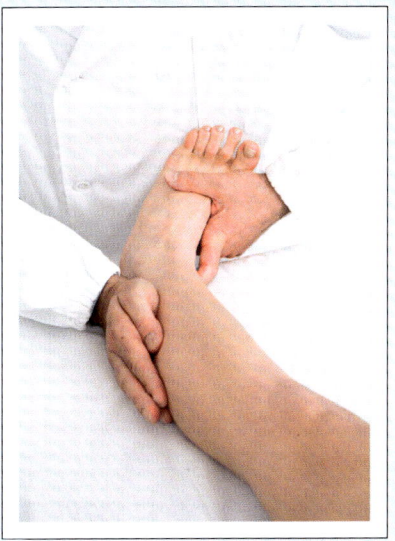

Dorsiflexion of toes is allowed.

PRONATOR QUADRATUS

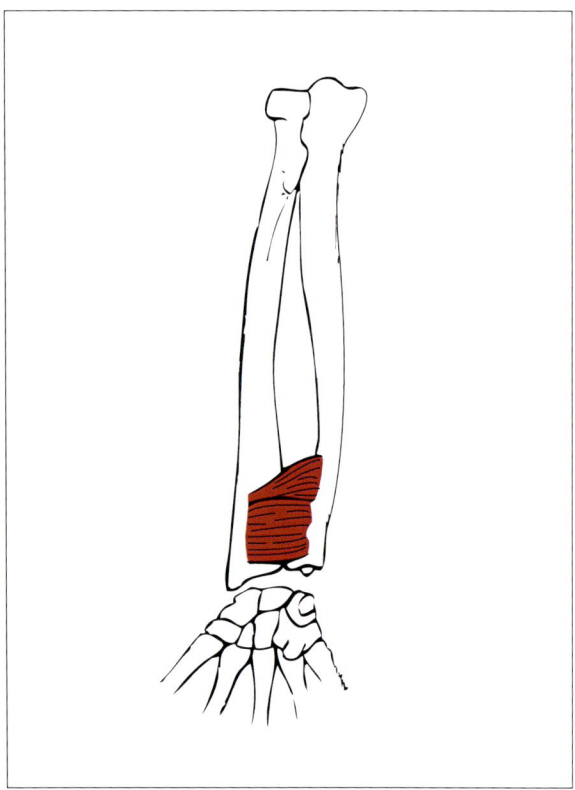

Pronator Quadratus
Origin: distal fourth of anterior surface of ulna.

Insertion: distal fourth of anterior surface of radius.

Innervation: median (C7-T1).

Action: pronates forearm; binds radius and ulna together.

CLINICAL*

- difficulty using a screwdriver
- carpal tunnel syndrome
- can't tolerate pressure on hands with wrist extension (i.e., push-ups, leaning on hands, etc.)
- wrist subluxations
- any wrist pain
- large intestine/stomach

*Courtesy of Drs. Walter Schmitt and Kerry McCord
Quintessential Applications: A(K) Clinical Protocol (QA)

PRONATOR QUADRATUS

Test 1

Position
Best tested seated, can be performed supine.

Test
Patient maximally flexes and pronates forearm. Examiner uses one hand to stabilize the elbow, while the other hand clasps the lateral surface of the distal forearm without causing pain, and directs pressure toward supination.

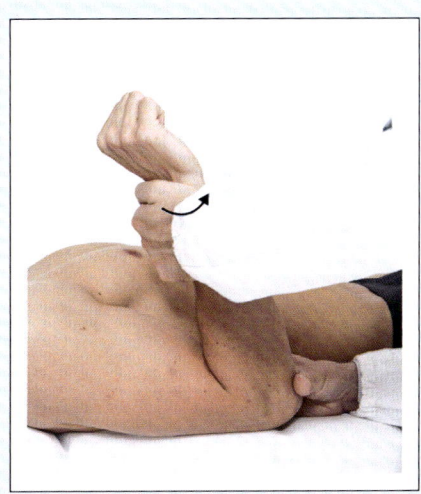
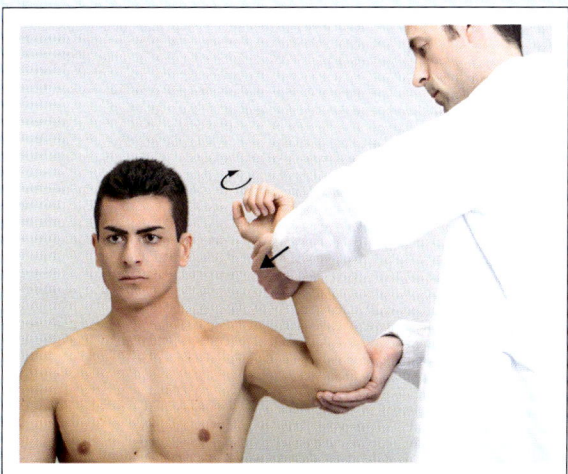

Test 2

Position
Best tested seated, can be performed supine.

Test
With the elbow locked in extension, patient abducts and flexes humerus to about 45 degrees, then fully pronates forearm.
Examiner stabilizes the elbow with one hand, while the other hand clasps the distal forearm without causing pain and directs pressure toward supination. This test is also used to evaluate Pronator Teres.

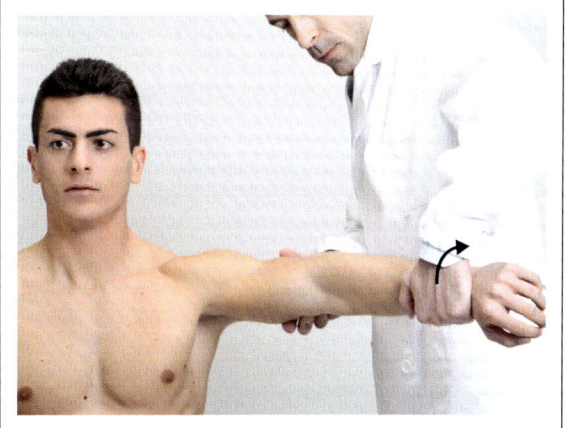

PRONATOR TERES

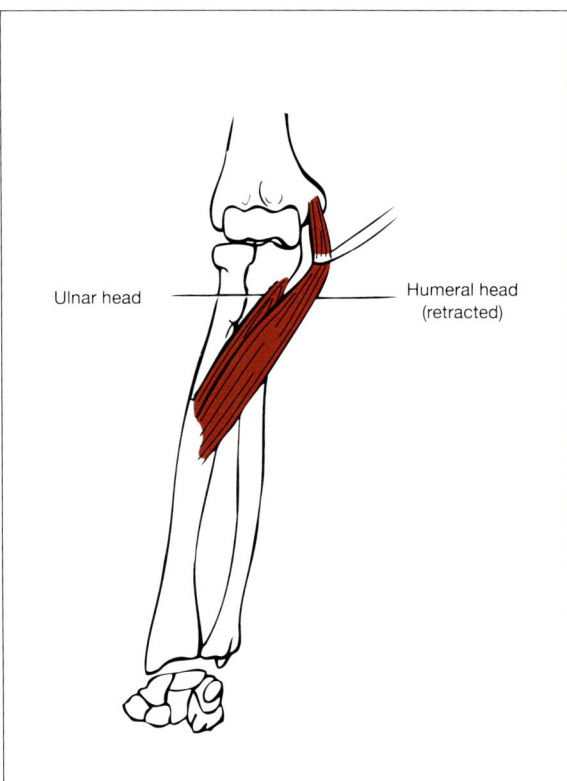

Pronator Teres

Origin humeral head: from the medial epicondylar ridge and common flexor tendon.

Origin ulnar head: medial surface of coronoid process of ulna.

Insertion: middle of lateral surface of radius.

Innervation: median (C6-C7).

Action: pronates forearm; flexes elbow joint.

Chapman's reflexes

1. **Anterior**: iliotibial band
   Posterior: L2 to L4 to crest of ilium

2. **Anterior**: anterior chest wall behind areola (not in breast tissue)
   Posterior: below inferior angle of scapula

Neurovascular point
lambdoidal suture midway between lambda and asterion

Acupuncture meridian association
stomach or large intestine (controversial)

Common subluxations
C5, C6

Associated point
T12, L1 (stomach or large intestine)

Visceral association
stomach or large intestine (controversial)

CLINICAL*

- difficulty/pain using a screwdriver
- elbow pain
- medial epicondylitis (golf elbow)
- radius subluxations
- wrist pain especially on pronation
- wrist subluxations
- stomach

*Courtesy of Drs. Walter Schmitt and Kerry McCord
Quintessential Applications: A(K) Clinical Protocol (QA)

PRONATOR TERES

Test 1

Position
Seated or supine.

Test
Patient flexes forearm to 60 degrees then fully pronates it. Examiner stabilizes posterior, distal humerus with one hand, while the other clasps the distal forearm without causing pain and directs pressure toward supination.

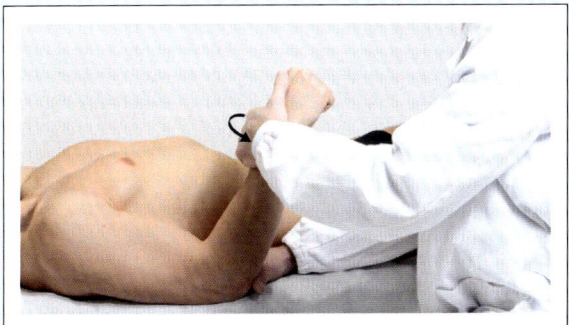

Common error

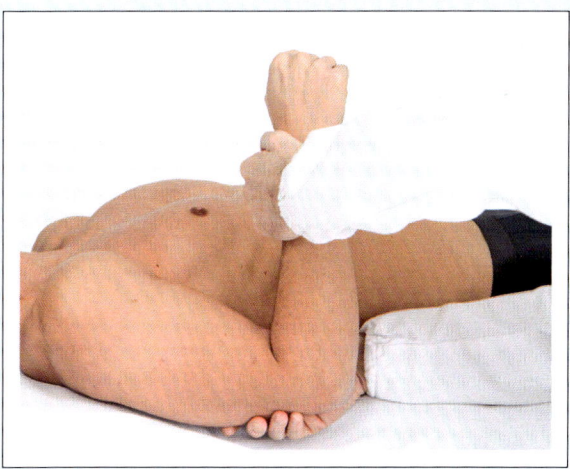

Excess forearm flexion.

Test 2

Position
Seated or supine.

Test
With the elbow locked in extension, patient abducts and flexes humerus to about 45 degrees then fully pronates forearm. Examiner stabilizes the elbow with one hand, while the other hand clasps the distal forearm without causing pain and directs pressure toward supination. It is impossible to exclude the Pronator Quadratus from this test.

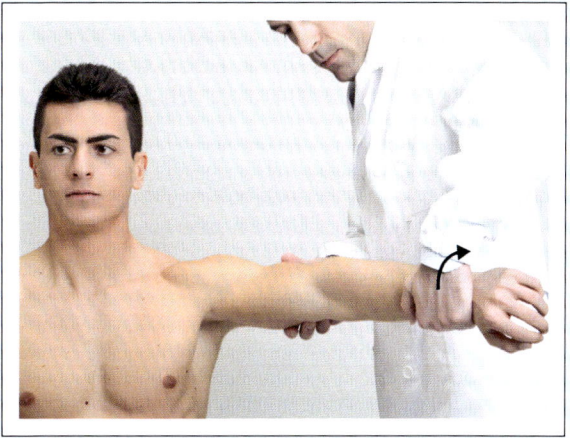

QUADRATUS LUMBORUM

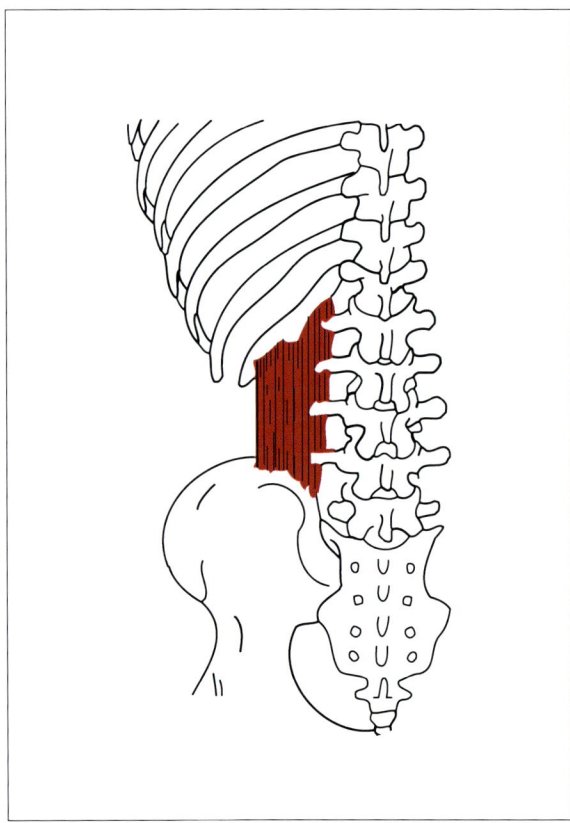

Quadratus Lumborum
Origin: iliolumbar ligament; posterior iliac crest.

Insertion: inferior border of rib 12; transverse processes of L1-L4.

Innervation: lumbar plexus (T12-L3).

Action: laterally flexes lumbar spine; depresses rib 12; assists diaphragm in inspiration.

Chapman's reflexes
Posterior 1: tip of rib 12
Posterior 2: T11

Neurovascular point
parietal eminence

Nutrition
vitamins A, C, and E

Acupuncture meridian association
large intestine

Meric TS line
L2

Common subluxations
T12-L3

Associated point
L4 and L5 (large intestine)

Visceral association
appendix

CLINICAL*

- low back pain often related to origin and insertion injury from trauma
- elevated rib 12 as seen on x-ray

*Courtesy of Drs. Walter Schmitt and Kerry McCord Quintessential Applications: A(K) Clinical Protocol (QA)

QUADRATUS LUMBORUM

Test

Position
Supine.

Test
With teeth lightly clenched, supine patient uses both hands to stabilize himself by clasping either side of the table. Then with the knees locked in extension and the legs aligned with the pelvis, the lumbar spine and pelvis are flexed laterally, toward the side being tested. Examiner is positioned on the opposite of that being tested, bent down low enough so that his trunk is level with the patient. One hand is used to stabilize at the ipsilateral, lateral pelvis while the other hand reaches under the legs distally to clasp the lateral surface of the contralateral leg. Both legs are then used as levers to impart force on the lumbar spine and pelvis, as examiner pulls toward himself, in the direction of ipsilateral, lateral flexion.

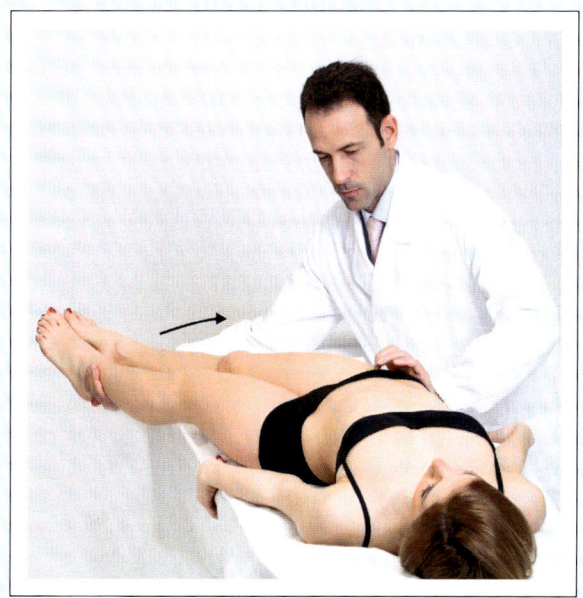

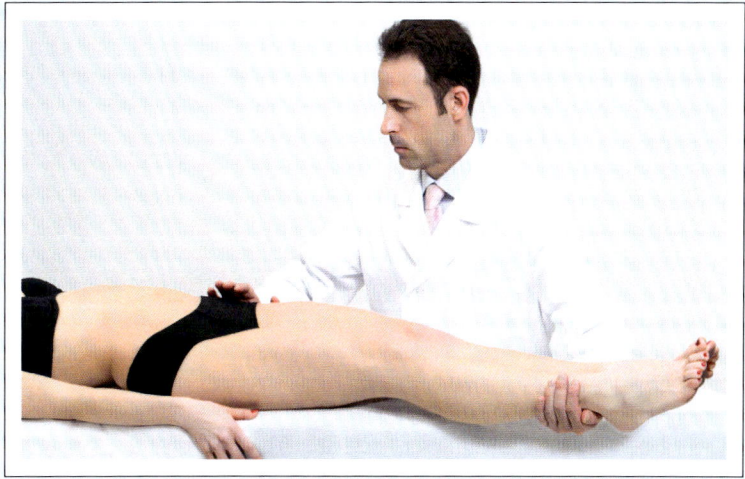

QUADRICEPS

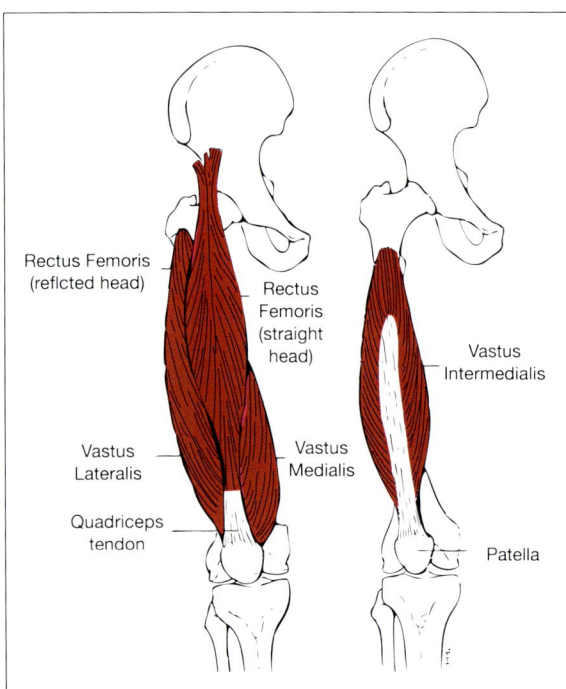

The quadriceps muscles consist of Rectus Femoris, Vastus Lateralis, Vastus Medialis, and Vastus Intermedius.

Rectus Femoris
Origin straight head: anterior inferior iliac spine.
Origin reflected head: groove superior to acetabulum.
Insertion: superior border of patella and via patellar ligament to tibial tuberosity.
Action: extends leg (knee) and flexes thigh (hip).

Vastus Intermedius
Origin: proximal three-fourths of the anterolateral surface of femur; lower half of linea aspera; upper part of lateral supracondylar line; lateral intermuscular septum.
Insertion: the superior border of patella and via patellar ligament to the tibial tuberosity.
Action: extends leg.

Vastus Medialis
Origin: inferior half of intertrochanteric line; medial lip of linea aspera; medial supracondylar line; medial intermuscular septum; tendons of adductor magnus and adductor longus.
Insertion: medial border of patella and via patellar ligament to tibial tuberosity.
Action: extends leg and draws patella medially.

Vastus Lateralis
Origin: greater trochanter; intertrochanteric line; gluteal tuberosity; linea aspera; lateral intermuscular septum; capsule of hip joint.
Insertion: lateral border of patella and via patellar ligament to tibial tuberosity.
Action: extends leg and draws patella laterally.

CLINICAL*
Quadriceps as a group

- difficulty going up stairs (especially after a meal)
- lateral or medial patella displacement (knee tracking problems)
- any knee problems
- when weak, stands with hyperextended knee or slightly flexed knee
- relaxed in knee extension ("locking home")
- articularis genu origin insertion pain (suprapatellar area)
- small intestine (food allergies)
- vitamin D

*Courtesy of Drs. Walter Schmitt and Kerry McCord
Quintessential Applications: A(K) Clinical Protocol (QA)

QUADRICEPS

The following applies to Rectus Femoris, Vastus Lateralis, Vastus Medialis, and Vastus Intermedius:

Innervation femoral (L2-L4)

Chapman's reflexes
Anterior: along lower border of rib cage, xyphoid to mid-mammilary line
Posterior: T8-T11

Neurovascular point
parietal eminences

Nutrition
vitamin D; vitamin B-complex; small intestine substance

Acupuncture meridian association
small intestine

Common subluxations
L2, L3, and L4

Meric TS line Rectus Femoris
T10

Meric TS line Vastus muscles
T12

Associated point
sacrum S1 and sacroiliac joint (small intestine)

Visceral association
small intestine

POSTURE

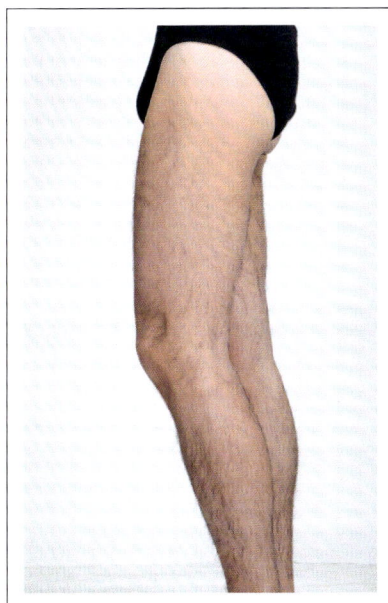
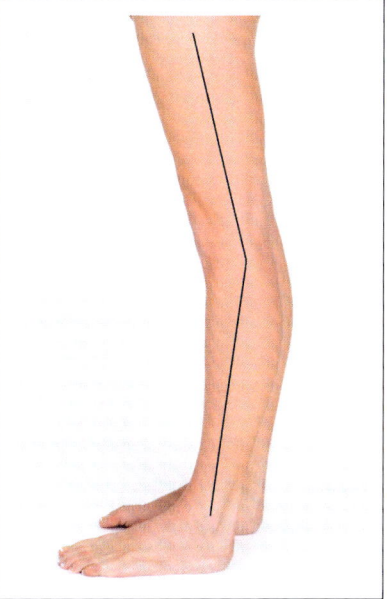

Quadriceps as a group: stands with flexed knee or knee in hyperextension.

QUADRICEPS

CLINICAL*
Rectus Femoris

- low back pain
- hip pain
- pain or weakness at origin (AIIS) on hip flexion ("hip pointer")
- knee pain (along with other quadriceps)

*Courtesy of Drs. Walter Schmitt and Kerry McCord
Quintessential Applications: A(K) Clinical Protocol (QA)

Rectus Femoris Test

Supine test
Patient flexes leg to 90 degrees, and femur to approximately 80 degrees. Examiner contacts the anterior distal femur and directs pressure toward extension.

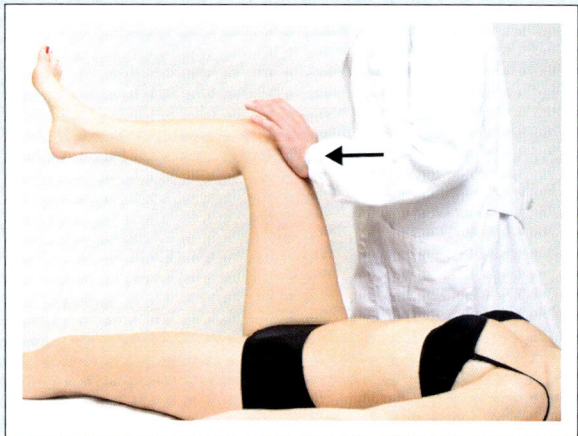

Alternate supine test
With teeth slightly clenched, patient fully extends leg and flexes femur to approximately 45 degrees. Examiner contacts the anterior surface of the distal leg and uses it as a lever by pushing downward toward the table to impart pressure toward femur extension.

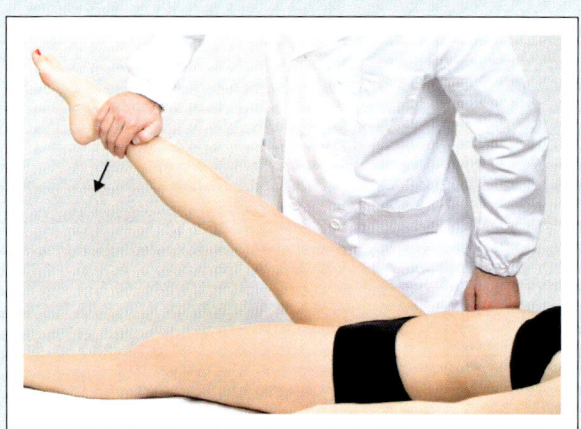

POSTURE

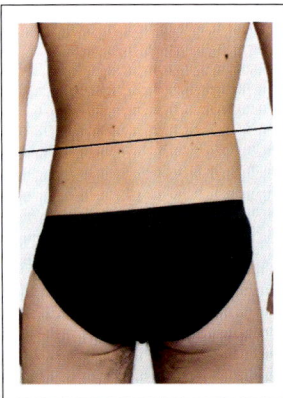

Rectus Femoris unilateral weakness: ipsilateral hip elevation.

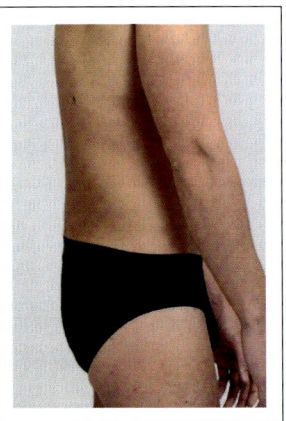

Rectus Femoris bilateral weakness: allows the superior portion of the pelvis to tilt posteriorly, creating lumbar hypolordosis.

QUADRICEPS

Rectus Femoris Test

Position
Seated or supine.

Seated test
With teeth lightly clenched, patient sits upright toward the edge of the table, knees and hips flexed to 90 degrees and hands on the table. Examiner contacts the anterior, distal femur and directs pressure toward thigh extension.

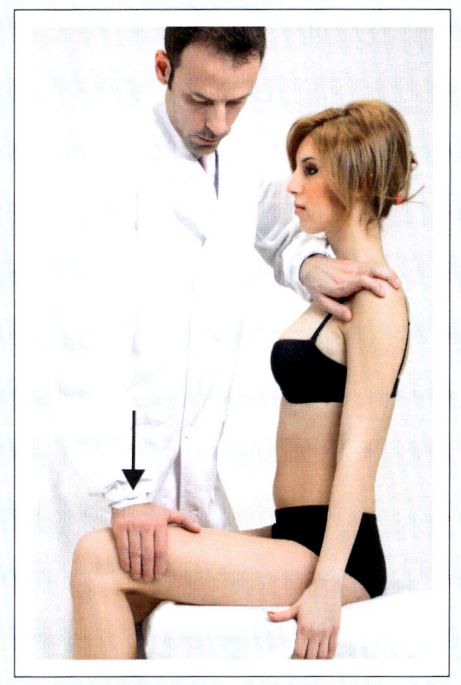

Common errors

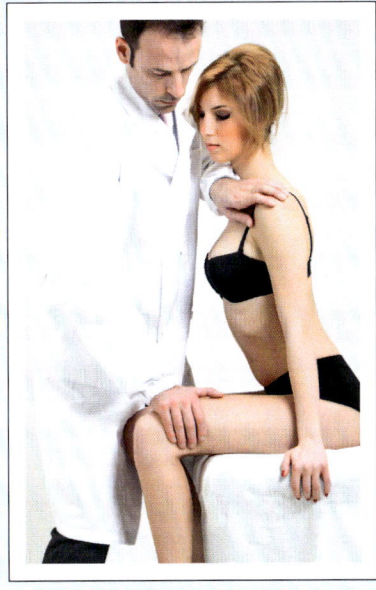

Patient is allowed to bend forward.

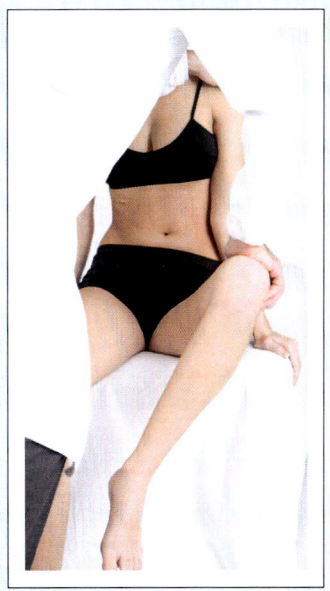

Femur is allowed to externally rotate and recruit iliopsoas.

QUADRICEPS

Vastus Intermedius Test

Position
Best performed supine, can be done seated.

Test
Patient lies supine with teeth lightly clenched, legs bent at the knees and hips, and feet planted on table. Examiner stands on the side being tested and reaches under the knee to place hand over the contralateral knee for leverage and stability. With the leg to be tested now resting on the examiner's forearm, patient extends leg to about 70 degrees. Examiner contacts the anterior surface of the distal leg and directs pressure toward flexion.

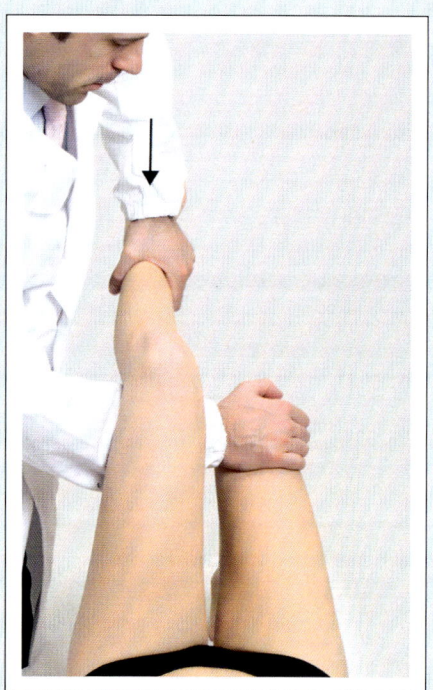

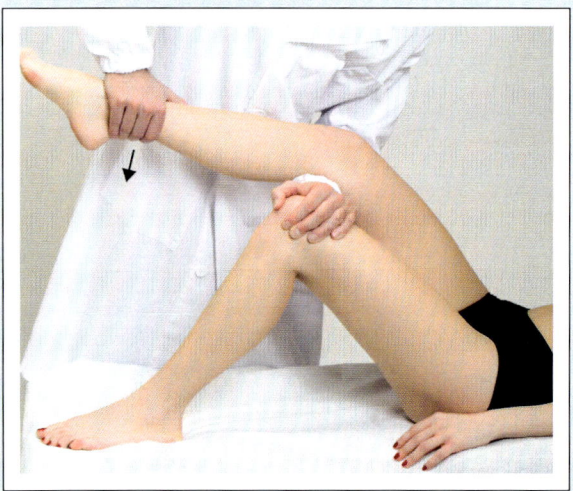

Common error

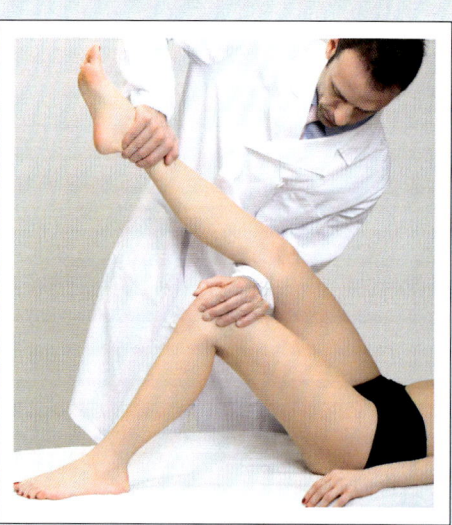

Too much leg extension.

QUADRICEPS

Vastus Medialis Test

Position
Best performed supine, can be done seated.

Test
Patient lies supine with teeth lightly clenched, legs bent at the knees and hips, and feet planted on table. Examiner stands on the side being tested and reaches under the knee to place hand over the contralateral knee in order to create leverage and stability. With the leg to be tested now resting on the examiner's forearm, patient medially rotates and extends leg to about 70 degrees. Examiner contacts the anterior surface of the distal leg, and directs pressure toward flexion and abduction (down and out).

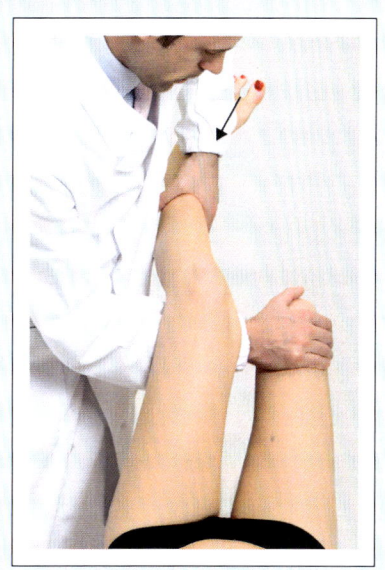

Vastus Lateralis Test

Position
Best performed supine, can be done seated.

Test
Patient lies supine with teeth lightly clenched, legs bent at the knees and hips, and feet planted on table. Examiner stands on the side being tested and reaches under the knee to place hand on the contralateral, distal femur for leverage and stability. With the leg to be tested now resting on the examiner's forearm, patient laterally rotates and extends leg to about 70 degrees. Examiner then contacts the anterior surface of the distal leg and directs pressure toward flexion and adduction (down and in).

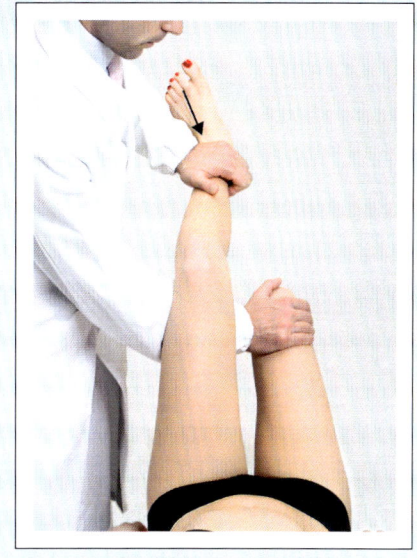

RHOMBOIDS

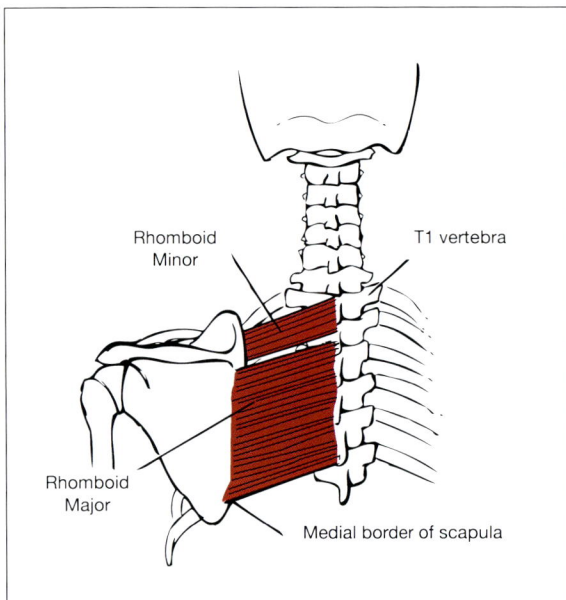

The Rhomboid muscles are divided into Rhomboid Minor and Rhomboid Major. In muscle testing they are tested as a unit.

Rhomboid Minor
Origin: spinous processes of C7 and T1.

Insertion: medial border of scapula (at the root of the spine of the scapula).

Innervation: dorsal scapular (C4-C5).

Action: adducts and slightly elevates scapula.

Rhomboid Major
Origin: spinous processes of T2-T5.

Insertion: medial border of scapula (from the root of the spine of the scapula to the inferior border).

Innervation: dorsal scapular nerve (C4-C5).

Action: retracts scapula and fixes scapula to thoracic wall; the inferior fibers aid in rotating glenoid cavity inferiorly.

Chapman's reflexes
Anterior: left 5th and 6th intercostal spaces
Posterior: left T5, T6, and T7

Neurovascular point
frontal bone eminences

Nutrition
vitamin A

Acupuncture meridian association
liver (or stomach-controversial)

Common subluxations
C4 and C5

Visceral association
liver (or stomach-controversial)

CLINICAL*

- woodsman swinging axe
- tight when antagonist is weak: i.e., serratus anterior, pectoralis major clavicular and pectoralis major sternal muscles

*Courtesy of Drs. Walter Schmitt and Kerry McCord Quintessential Applications: A(K) Clinical Protocol (QA)

RHOMBOIDS

POSTURE

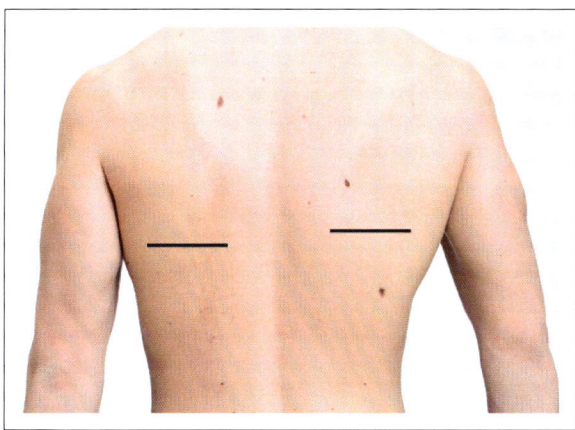

Scapula will sag and head may rotate toward side of weakness.

Test

Position
Best tested seated, can also be tested with patient side-lying.

Test
Seated patient lightly clenches teeth and abducts non-tested arm to above 90 degrees in order to prevent recruiting opposite rhomboid. The humerus of the side being tested is held in adduction with 90 degrees forearm flexion. Examiner stabilizes ipsilateral shoulder with one hand while the other contacts the medial surface of the distal humerus and directs pressure toward abduction. During the test, examiner observes scapula for abduction (away from spine) which would indicate a positive test.

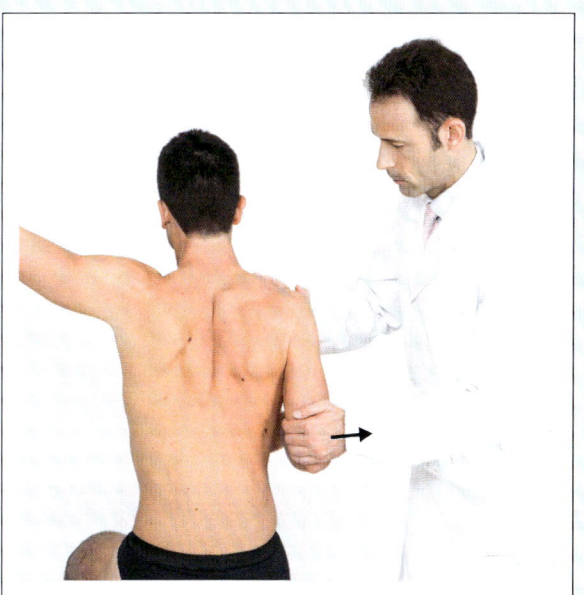

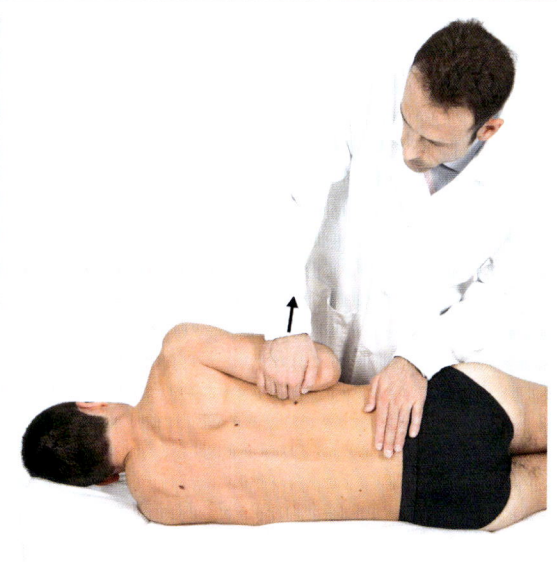

SACROSPINALIS
ERECTOR SPINAE

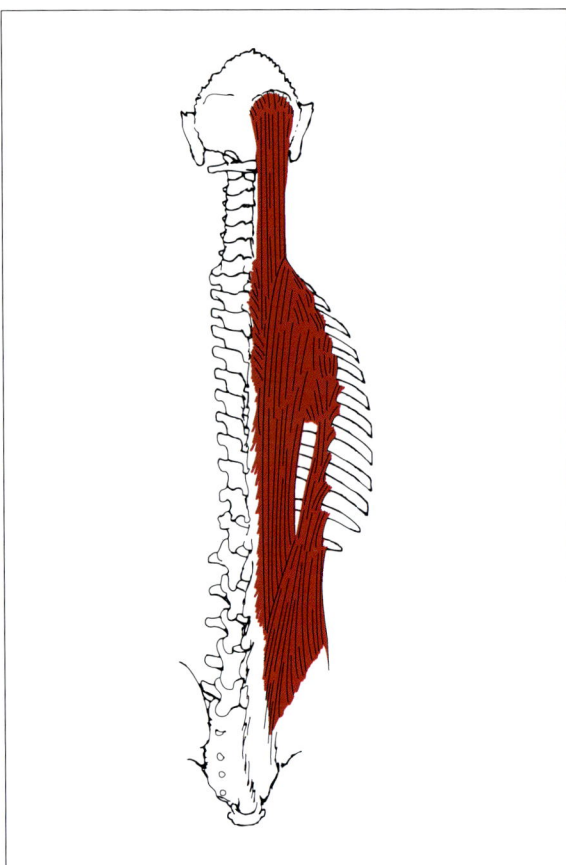

Sacrospinalis (Erector Spinae)

Origin: the sacrospinalis is not just one muscle, but a bundle of muscles and tendons that originate at the sacrum, crest of ilium, spinous processes, transverse processes, and ribs.

Insertion: ribs; transverse processes; spinous processes; occiput.

Innervation: various.

Action: extension, lateral flexion, and ipsilateral rotation and lateral flexion of spinal column.

Chapman's reflexes
Anterior: lateral to umbillicus; symphysis pubis
Posterior: L2

Neurovascular point
frontal bone eminences

Nutrition
vitamins A, C, E; bioflavinoids (vitamin P)

Acupuncture meridian association
bladder

Common subluxations
various, especially lower sacrum

Associated point
sacrum S2 (bladder)

Visceral association
bladder

CLINICAL*

- "C" spine curve convex on tight side the opposite side of weakness
- difficulty in lateral bending or difference in right and left lateral bending
- tight side is visible or palpable with patient prone: muscle is "bunched up"

*Courtesy of Drs. Walter Schmitt and Kerry McCord Quintessential Applications: A(K) Clinical Protocol (QA)

SACROSPINALIS ERECTOR SPINAE

POSTURE

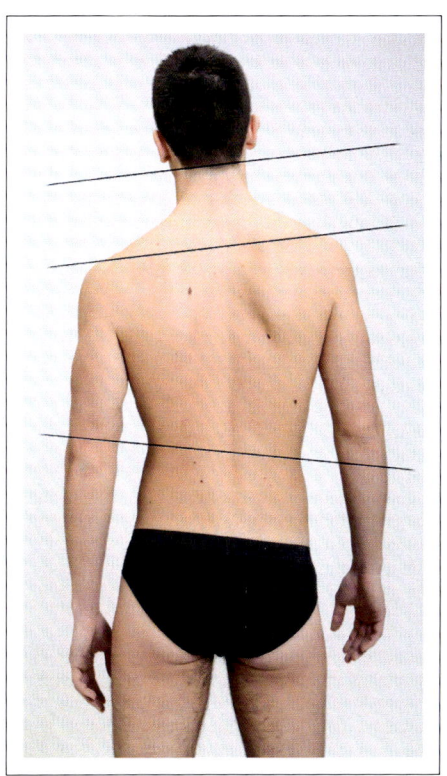

"C" curve of spinal column, convex on weak side.

Test 1

Position
Standing.

Test
Patient stands barefoot, with feet shoulders' width apart, then laterally flexes the trunk, reaching down the leg as far as possible as examiner observes from behind. The same movement is then repeated on the opposite side while examiner observes and compares. The patient will be able to laterally flex farther on the side opposite of weakness. All factors that may influence the outcome of this test must be considered: spinal curvatures, leg length inequality, muscle weakness of Quadratus Lumborum, Iliopsoas, Abdominals, and Latissimus Dorsi.

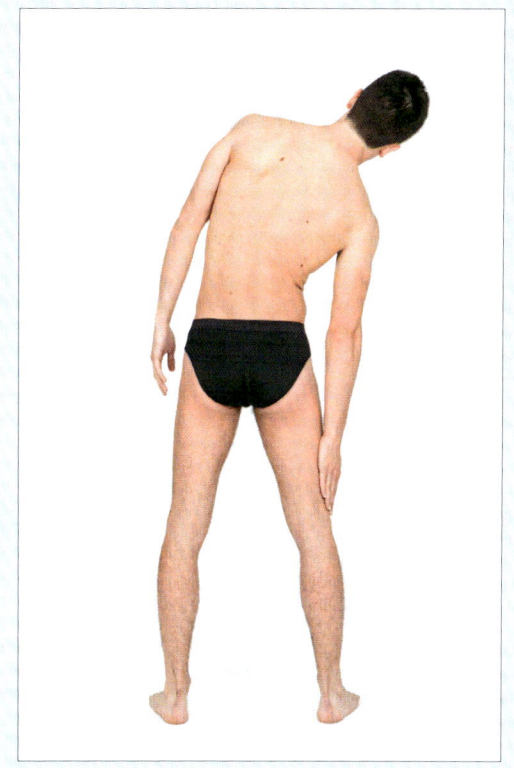

SACROSPINALIS ERECTOR SPINAE

Test 2

Position
Prone.

Test
With arms at sides and inactive, prone patient hyperextends and rotates the spine toward the side being tested. Examiner stands on same side and uses one hand to stabilize over the posterior contralateral ilium, while the other hand makes a flat contact over the ipsilateral scapula and directs pressure toward flexion and contralateral rotation of the spine (back down toward the table). This is a general test, and synergists must be considered.

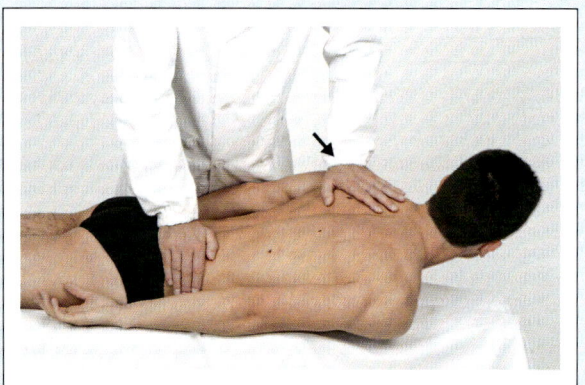

Common error

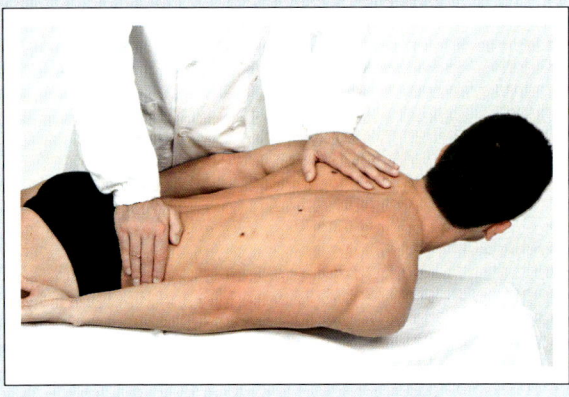

Examiner pushes straight down toward the table.

SARTORIUS

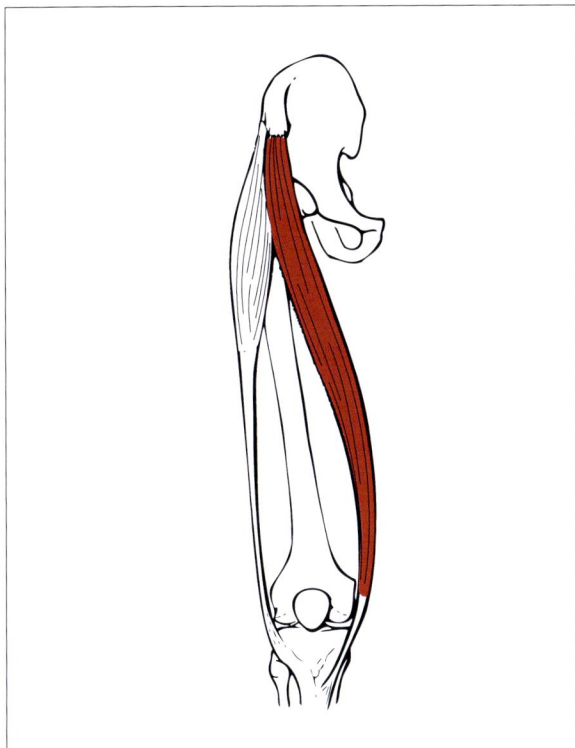

Sartorius

Origin: anterior superior iliac spine; superior part of iliac notch.

Insertion: pes anserinus; superior part of medial surface of tibia.

Innervation: femoral nerve (L2-L4).

Action: flexes tibia; abducts, flexes, and externally rotates femur; internally rotates tibia when knee is flexed; gives medial support to knee.

Chapman's reflexes
Anterior: 1 inch lateral and 2 inches superior to umbillicus
Posterior: T11 and T12

Neurovascular point
lambda

Nutrition
adrenal substance; vitamin C; pantothenic acid; niacinamide; wheat germ oil; DHEA; adaptogens

Acupuncture meridian association
circulation sex (pericardium)

Common subluxations
L2, L3 and L4

Meric TS line
T9

Associated point
T4 and T5 (circulation sex)

Visceral association
adrenals

CLINICAL*

- any knee problems
- medial meniscus injury
- difficulty (especially at medial knee) going down stairs
- pain at origin "hip pointer"
- iliotibial band tightness
- tripod muscle: knee and pelvic stabilization
- category 2 posterior ilium (UoMS)
- adrenals

*Courtesy of Drs. Walter Schmitt and Kerry McCord
Quintessential Applications: A(K) Clinical Protocol (QA)

SARTORIUS

POSTURE

Genu valgus ("knock knees");
pelvic posterior rotation on weak side.

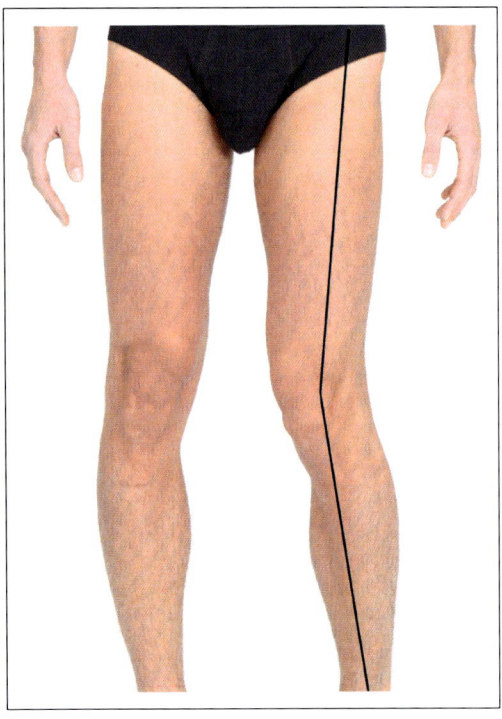

Test

Position
Supine.

Test
With teeth lightly clenched, supine patient flexes leg (knee) to 90 degrees, while externally rotating, abducting, and flexing the femur to position the foot over the opposite knee (figure 4 configuration). During the test, some patients will seek to compensate a weak sartorius by medially rotating the femur, while others will tend toward lateral rotation. Therefore, the position of the examiner's stabilization hand will vary: either over the anterior or the over the lateral surface of distal femur. The examiner's other hand grasps the posterior, distal leg around the achilles tendon. This is a two-joint test in which both hands apply pressure simultaneously: the hand on the femur directs pressure toward extension, adduction, and internal rotation, while the hand on the leg pulls toward extension.

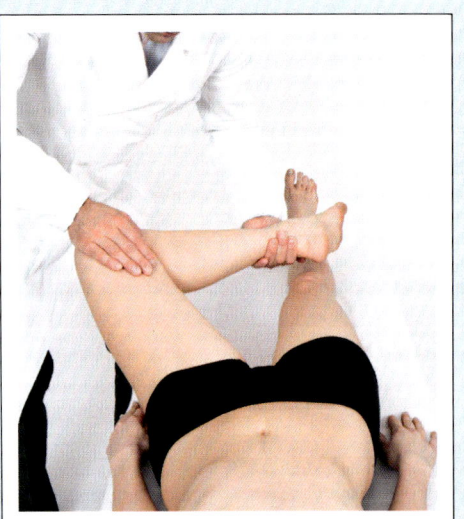
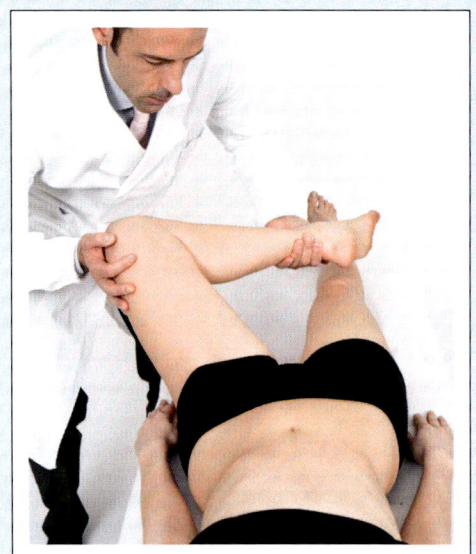

SARTORIUS

Test

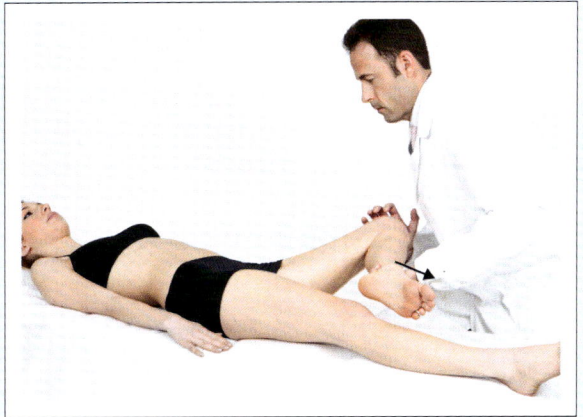 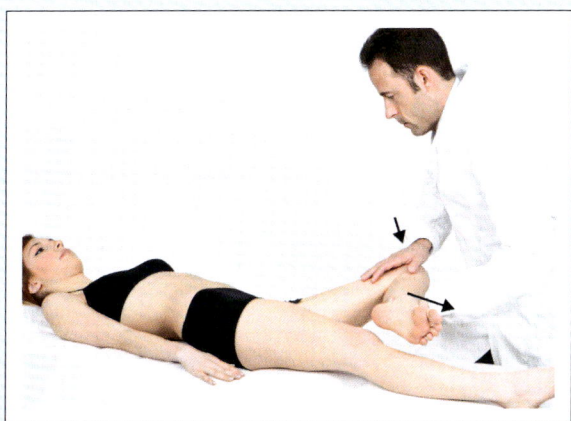

The position of the examiner's stabilizing hand may vary.

Common error

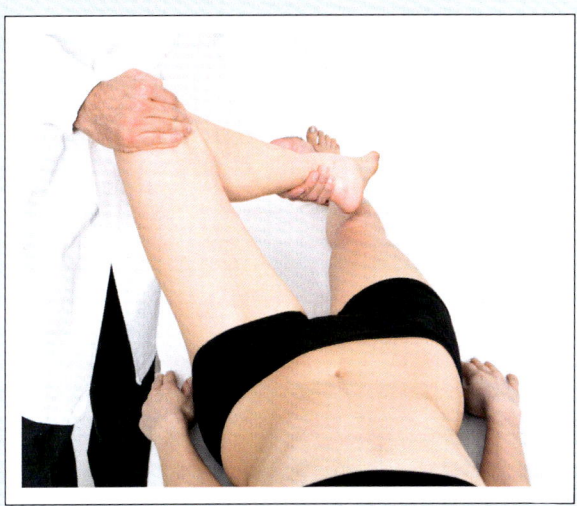

Lack of rotational test force allows hamstrings to be recruited.

SERRATUS ANTERIOR

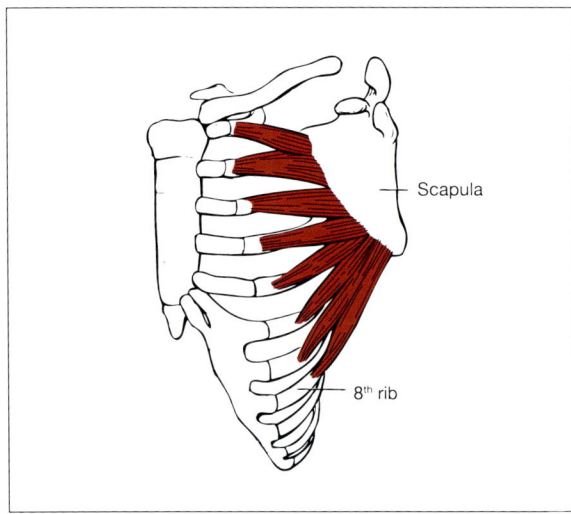

Serratus Anterior
Origin: external surfaces and superior borders of the lateral parts of ribs 1 to 8.

Insertion: costal surface of the vertebral border of scapula.

Innervation: long thoracic (C5-C7).

Action: abducts and rotates scapula to point glenoid cavity superiorly; assists in holding vertebral border of scapula against thoracic wall.

Chapman's reflexes
Anterior: 2nd, 3rd, 4th and 5th intercostal spaces
Posterior: T3, T4, and T5

Neurovascular point
bregma

Nutrition
vitamin C; lung substances

Acupuncture meridian association
lung

Common subluxations
C5, C6, and C7

Meric TS line
T3

Associated point
T3 and T4 (lung)

Visceral association
lungs

CLINICAL*

- in paralysis, humerus abduction limited to 90 degrees
- difficulty reaching or pushing forward
- when weak, ipsilateral rhomboids will be tight
- observe for scapular movement during abduction
- injured when catching self falling forward
- breathing problems related to diaphragm and/or rib positions
- breathing problems related to lungs
- pseudo-breast soreness from injuries to origins
- C7 to T2 A.K. fixations when weak bilaterally

*Courtesy of Drs. Walter Schmitt and Kerry McCord Quintessential Applications: A(K) Clinical Protocol (QA)

SERRATUS ANTERIOR

POSTURE

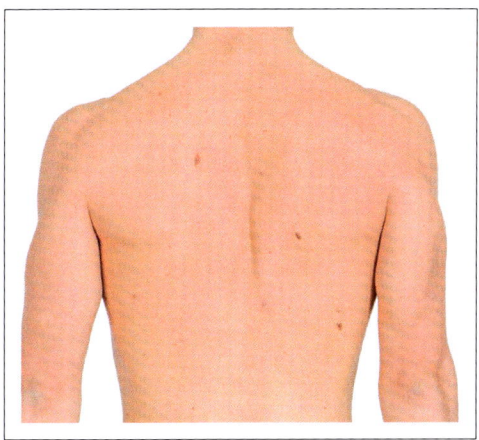

Winged scapula or tight ipsilateral rhomboid.

Test

Position
Best tested seated but can also be performed supine.

Test
With forearm locked at the elbow, patient abducts and flexes humerus to approximately 100-130 degrees (the amount of abduction and flexion is varied depending on which section of the muscle is being tested). Examiner contacts the lateral surface of the distal forearm with one hand, while the other hand is placed over the inferior, lateral border of the scapula. Using the forearm as a lever, examiner directs pressure toward extension and adduction of the humerus, in order to impart subsequent pressure toward adduction of the inferior angle of the scapula. As pressure is applied, examiner checks for adduction of the inferior angle of the scapula as this would indicate a positive test, whereas inability of the arm to resist test pressure would not.

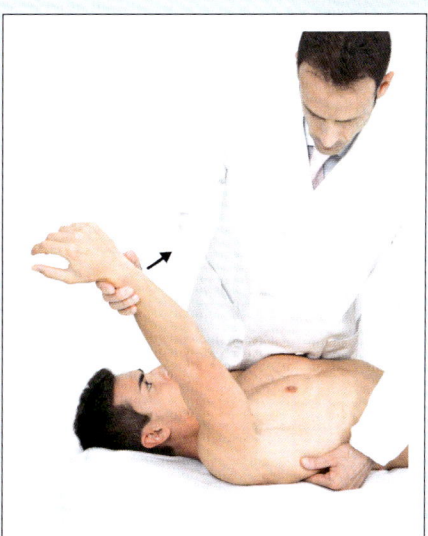
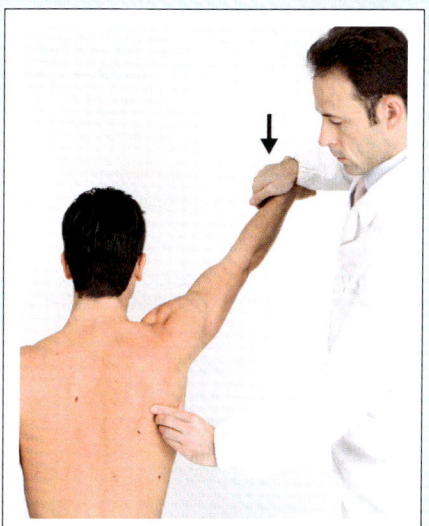

SERRATUS ANTERIOR

Test

The amount of abduction and flexion is varied depending on which section of the muscle is being tested.

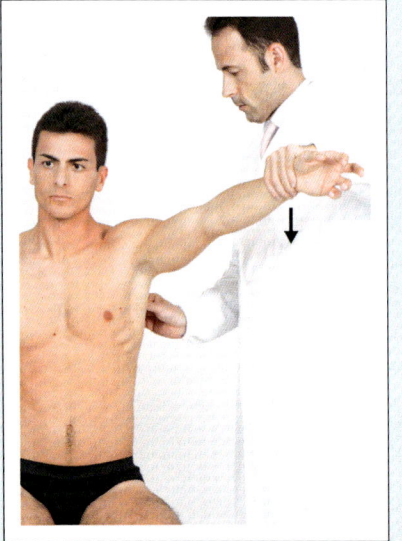
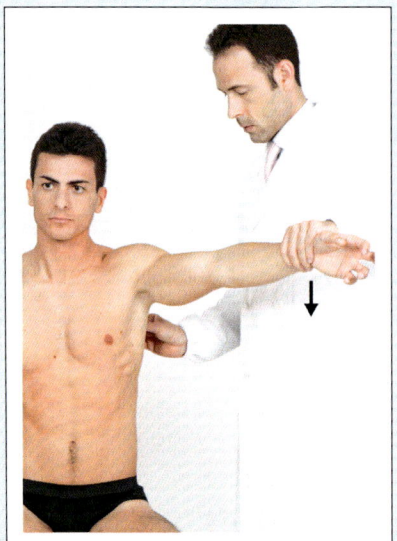
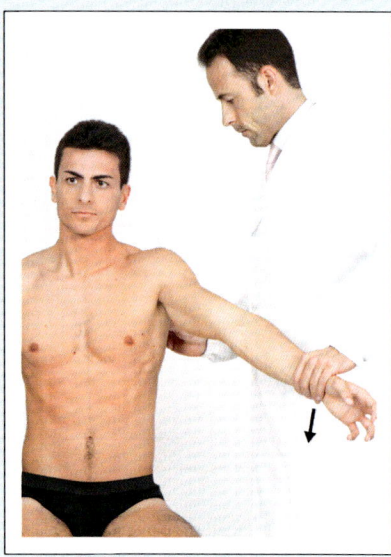

Common error

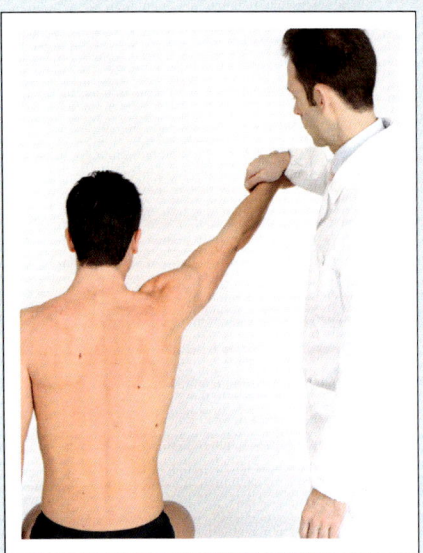

Examiner fails to palpate for scapular movement and concludes that the test is positive because the arm is unable to resist test pressure.

SOLEUS

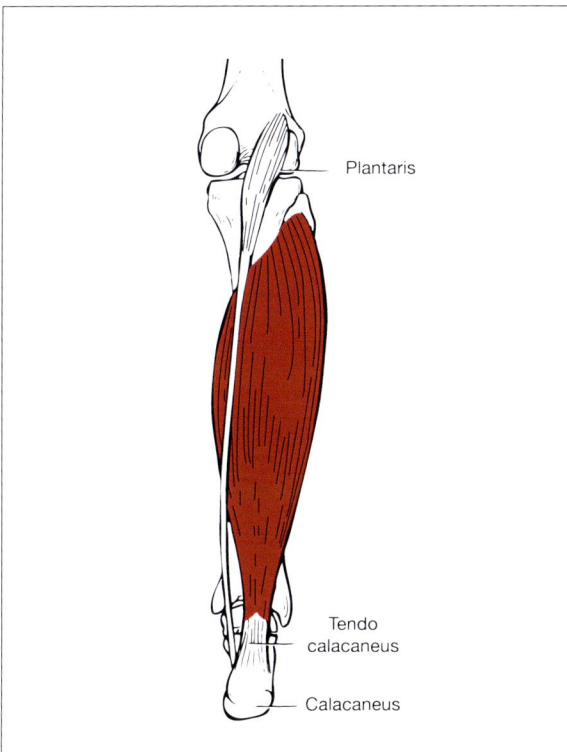

Soleus
Origin: posterior surface of head and superior third of the shaft of fibula; middle third of the medial border of tibia; tendinous arch between tibia and fibula.

Insertion: posterior surface of calcaneus.

Innervation: tibial (L4-S2).

Action: plantarflexes foot.

Chapman's reflexes
Anterior: 1 inch lateral and 2 inches superior to umbillicus
Posterior: T11 and T12

Neurovascular point
bregma

Nutrition
adrenal substance; vitamin C; pantothenic acid; niacinamide; wheat germ oil; DHEA; adaptogens.

Acupuncture meridian association
circulation sex (pericardium)

Common subluxations
L4-S2

Meric TS line
T9

Associated point
T4 and T5 (circulation sex)

Visceral association
adrenals

CLINICAL*

- powerful plantar flexor (gastrocnemeus is far less powerful)
- important in "take off" phase of walking, running or cycling
- difficulty standing up on tip toes (gets help from gastrocnemeus)
- recurrent calcaneus subluxations
- adrenals

*Courtesy of Drs. Walter Schmitt and Kerry McCord Quintessential Applications: A(K) Clinical Protocol (QA)

SOLEUS

POSTURE

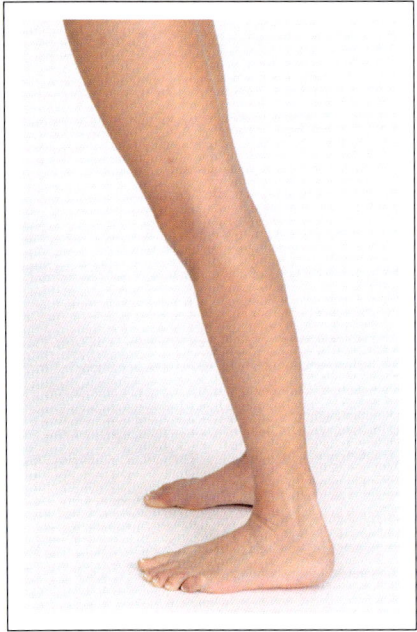

Forward lean.

Test

Position
Prone.

Test
Patient lightly clenches teeth, flexes knee to 90 degrees and maximally plantarflexes foot. Examiner clasps the posterior calcaneus with one hand, while the other clasps the plantar surface of the forefoot. Force is then directed through both hands simultaneously: tractional pressure at the posterior calcaneus, and dorsiflexion pressure at the forefoot.

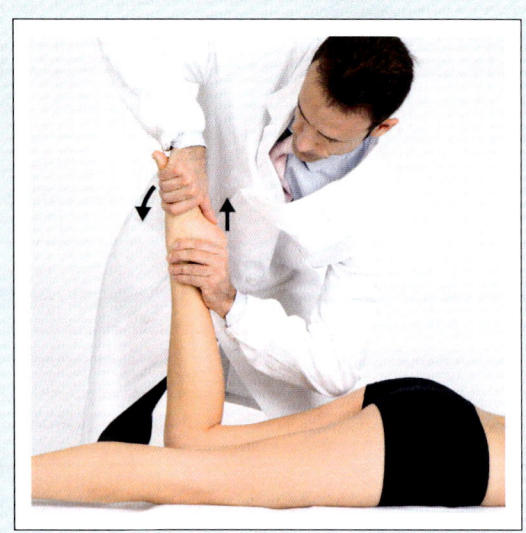

STERNOCLEIDOMASTOID

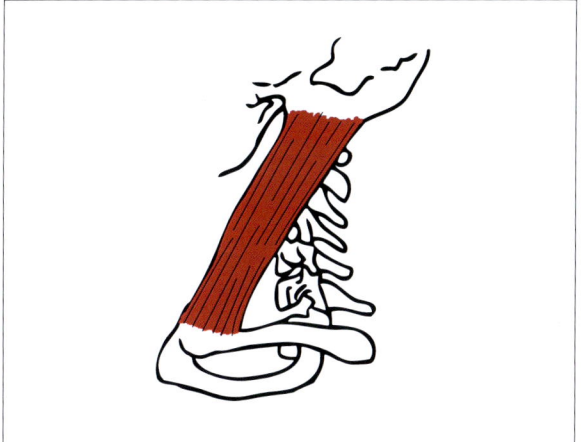

Sternocleidomastoid
Origin sternal head: anterior surface of manubrium lateral to jugular notch.
Origin clavicular head: upper surface of medial half of clavicle.

Insertion: lateral surface of mastoid process of temporal bone and the lateral half of the superior nuchal line of occipital bone.

Innervation: spinal root of accessory nerve (CN XI); anterior rami of C2 and C3.

Action: acting unilaterally, it laterally flexes neck by drawing mastoid process inferiorly toward ipsilateral shoulder, while simultaneously rotating the head contralaterally.
Acting bilaterally, the sternocleidomastoids flex the head and neck.

Chapman's reflexes
Anterior: inferior to mid-clavicle
Posterior: C0-C2 laminae

Neurovascular point
ramus of mandible

Nutrition
niacinamide or niacin with vitamin B6 (5:1 ratio); organic iodine for sinusitis

Acupuncture meridian association
stomach

Common subluxations
upper cervicals and cranial faults

Meric TS line
rib 1 and T1

Associated point
T12, L1 (stomach)

Visceral association
sinuses

CLINICAL*

- whiplash injury (origin and insertion injury)
- neck flexion/extension problems
- pain and limited range of motion with lateral flexion (i.e., holding phone to ear)
- pain and limited range of motion on neck rotation (i.e., rotating head while backing up car)
- frontal bone fault causes bilateral SCM weakness
- sinus problems

*Courtesy of Drs. Walter Schmitt and Kerry McCord Quintessential Applications: A(K) Clinical Protocol (QA)

STERNOCLEIDOMASTOID

Bilateral Sternocleidomastoids Test 1

Position
Seated or supine.

Test
Keeping the chin tucked, patient lifts head by maximally flexing neck and head while keeping the chin tucked. Examiner places one hand under the head to catch it should it suddenly fall back toward the table, while the other hand contacts the patient's forehead and directs pressure toward neck extension.

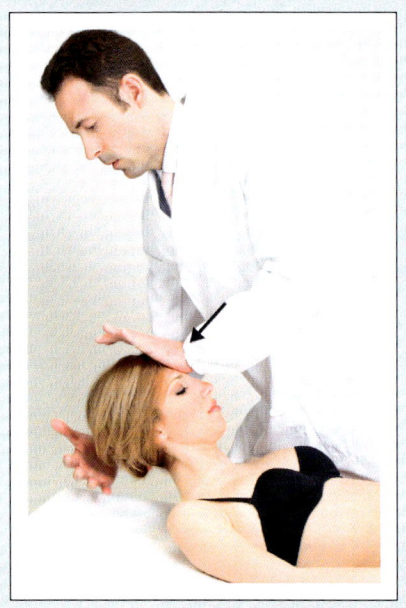

Bilateral Sternocleidomastoids Test 2

Position
Seated or supine.

Test
The test is repeated as above but with the patient's arms abducted to 90 degrees and forearms flexed to 90 degrees.

N.B.
Sometimes these muscles are only found to be weak when the arms are held above the head. Therefore, the test is performed first with the arms at the sides. Then, only if no weakness was found in this position, is the test repeated with the arms above the head.

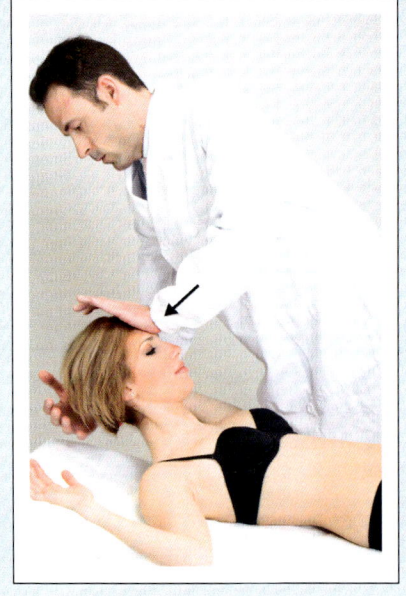

STERNOCLEIDOMASTOID

Unilateral Sternocleidomastoid Test 1

Position
Seated or supine.

Test
Patient rotates head away from the side being tested then maximally flexes neck to lift head off the table. Examiner places one hand under the head to catch it should it suddenly fall back toward the table, while the other hand contacts the parietal bone and directs pressure toward head and neck extension.

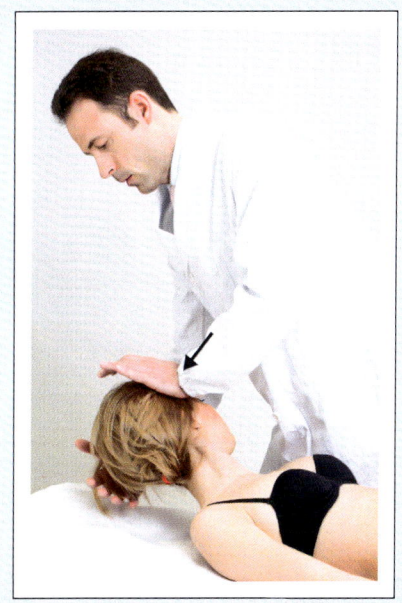

Unilateral Sternocleidomastoid Test 2

Position
Seated or supine.

Test
The test is repeated as above but with the patient's arms abducted to 90 degrees and forearms flexed to 90 degrees.

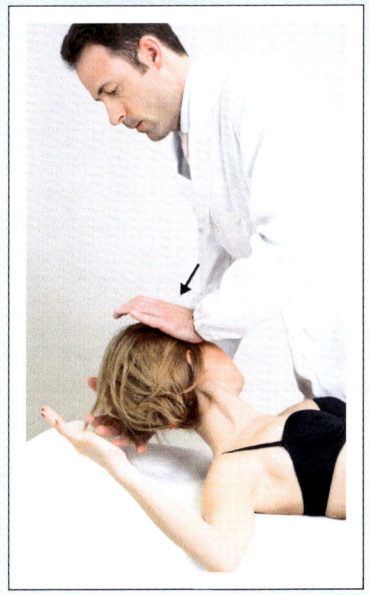

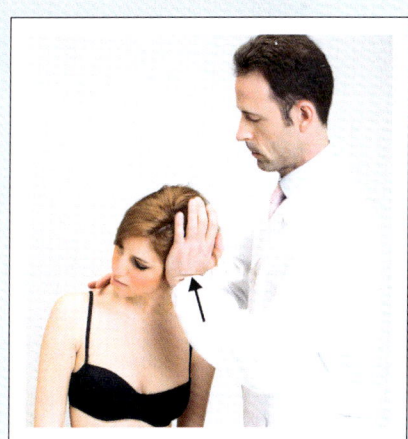

The test can also be performed in the seated position in which case it is not necessary to have patient raise the arms above the head.

135

STERNOCLEIDOMASTOID

Common errors

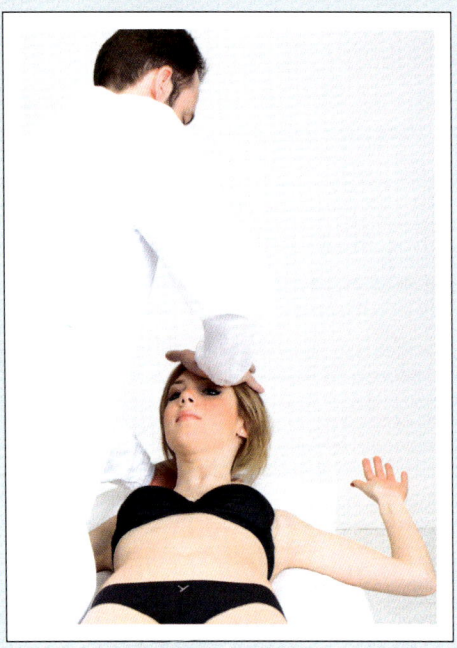

Patient's head is allowed to rotate back toward the midline.

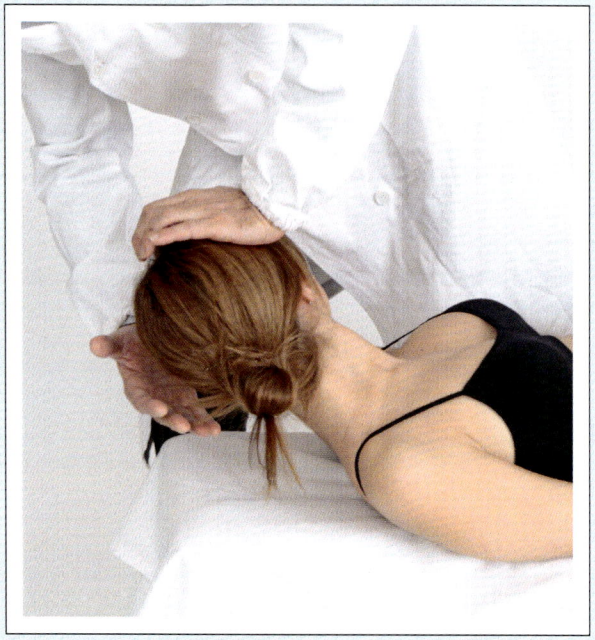

Pressure is directed straight down toward table instead of in a cephalad vector, in line with the fibers of the muscle.

SUBSCAPULARIS

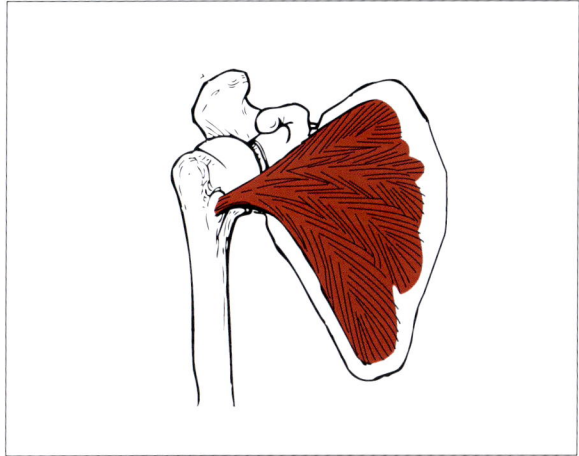

Subscapularis
Origin sternal head: subscapular fossa.

Insertion: lesser tubercle of humerus and capsule of shoulder joint.

Innervation: upper and lower subscapular (C5-C7).

Action: internally rotates humerus; draws head of humerus forward and down when elevated; assists in holding humeral head in glenoid cavity.

Chapman's reflexes
Anterior: 2nd intercostal space
Posterior: T2, T3

Neurovascular point
bregma

Nutrition
heart substance; vitamins A, C and B-complex (including "B" and "G")

Acupuncture meridian association
heart

Common subluxations
C5 and C6

Meric TS line
T2

Associated point
T5 and T6 (heart)

Visceral association
heart

CLINICAL*

- problems throwing
- difficulty playing tennis (forehand) or golf
- difficulty reaching forward
- difficulty reaching across body
- can't get arm up behind back
- origin and insertion injury in "rotator cuff syndrome"
- must consider entire origin in injury
- heart

*Courtesy of Drs. Walter Schmitt and Kerry McCord Quintessential Applications: A(K) Clinical Protocol (QA)

SUBSCAPULARIS

POSTURE

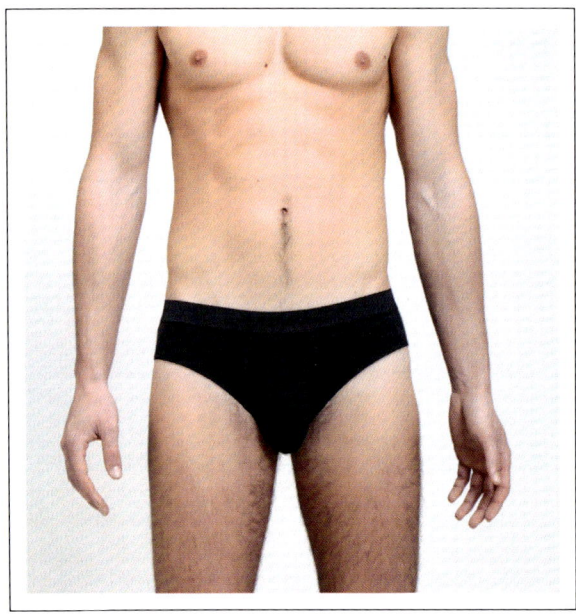

Arm, forearm and hand hang in external rotation. The palm will either face forward or in less extreme cases, the hand will rotate externally from the frontal plane.

Test

Position
Seated, supine or prone.

Test
In the supine and seated position, patient lightly clenches teeth, abducts humerus to 90 degrees, and flexes the forearm to 90 degrees. Then depending on the individual patient's anatomical shoulder formation, the humerus may be internally rotated anywhere in the range from zero to about 45 degrees. Examiner uses one hand to stabilize the posterior, distal humerus, while the other hand contacts the anterior, distal forearm and directs pressure toward external rotation of the humerus, using the forearm as a lever.

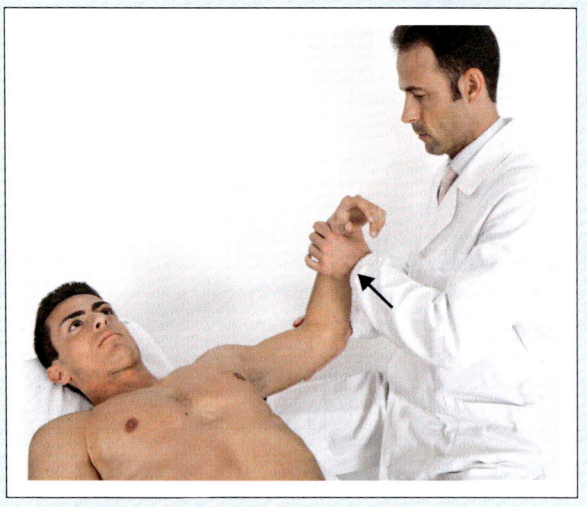

SUBSCAPULARIS

Test

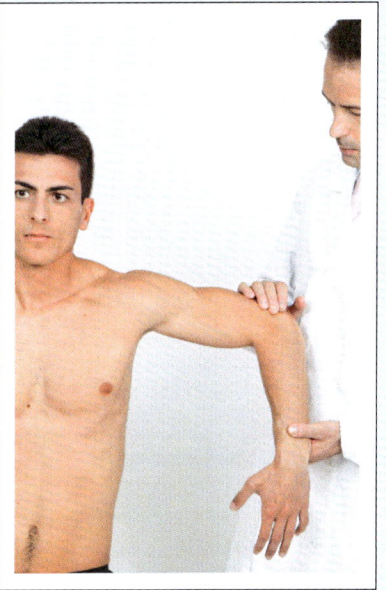
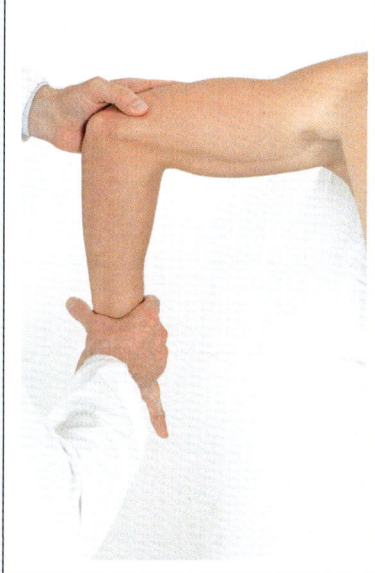
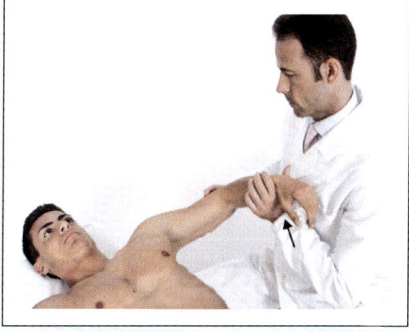

Alternate starting position.

Common errors

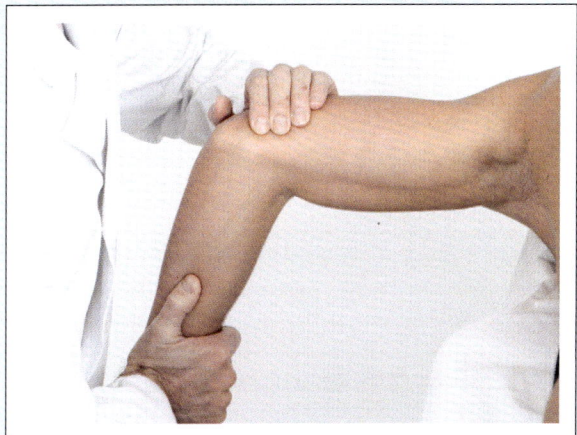

Too much elbow extension.

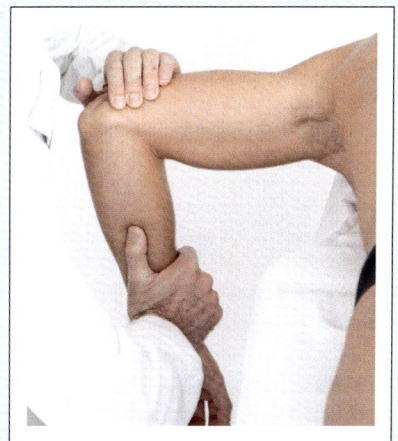

Too much elbow flexion.

SUPINATOR

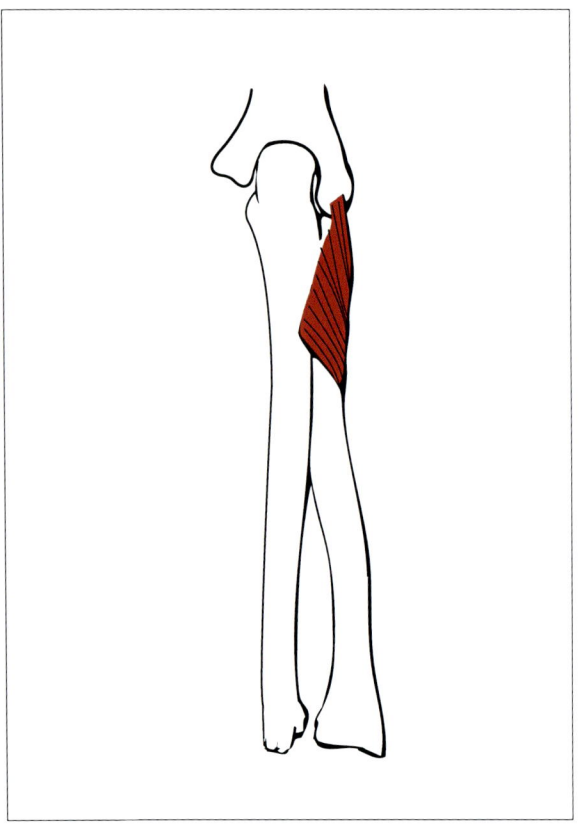

Supinator
Origin: lateral condyle of humerus; radial collateral ligament of elbow; annular ligaments of humerus; supinator fossa and crest of ulna.

Insertion: lateral, posterior, and anterior surfaces of proximal third or radius.

Innervation: radial (C5-C6).

Action: supinates forearm.

CLINICAL*

- pain/limited range of motion with forearm supination (e.g., using a screwdriver)
- any elbow problem

*Courtesy of Drs. Walter Schmitt and Kerry McCord Quintessential Applications: A(K) Clinical Protocol (QA)

Chapman's reflexes
Anterior: left 5th and 6th intercostal space
Posterior: left T5, T6, and T7

Neurovascular point
frontal bone eminences

Nutrition
vitamins "B," "G" and HCL

Acupuncture meridian association
stomach

SUPINATOR

Test 1

Position
Best tested seated, can be performed supine.

Test
With elbow locked in extension, patient abducts and flexes humerus to approximately 45 degrees, then fully supinates forearm. Examiner stabilizes the elbow with one hand while the other hand clasps the distal forearm without causing pain, and directs pressure toward pronation.

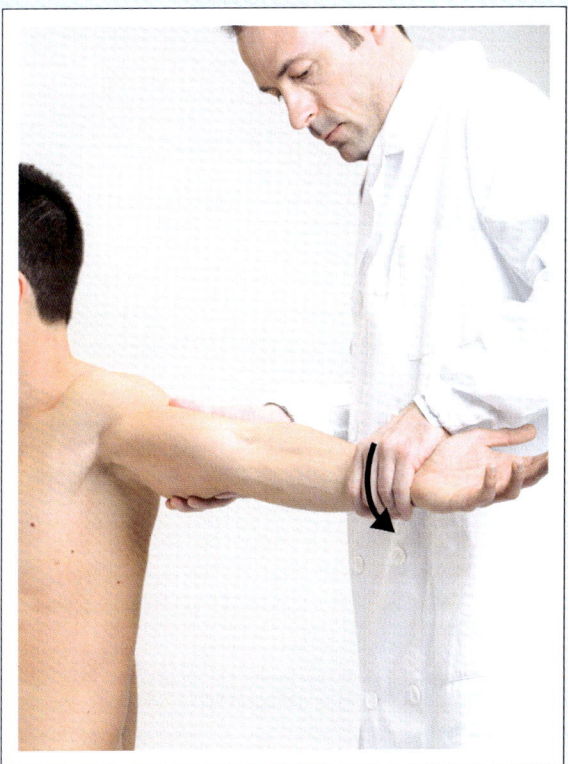

Test 2

Position
Best tested seated, can be performed supine.

Test
Patient flexes humerus to approximately 60 to 70 degrees then maximally flexes and supinates forearm. Examiner uses one hand to stabilize the elbow, while the other hand clasps the distal forearm without causing pain, and directs pressure toward pronation.

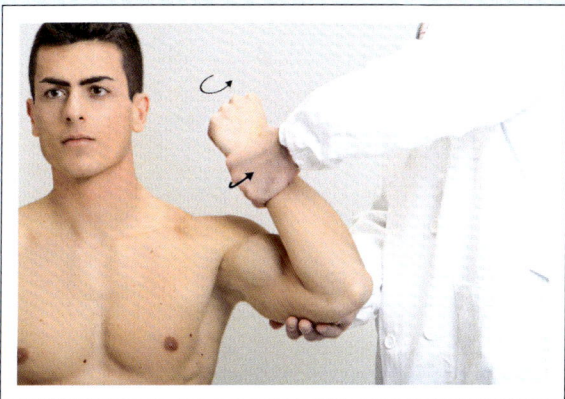

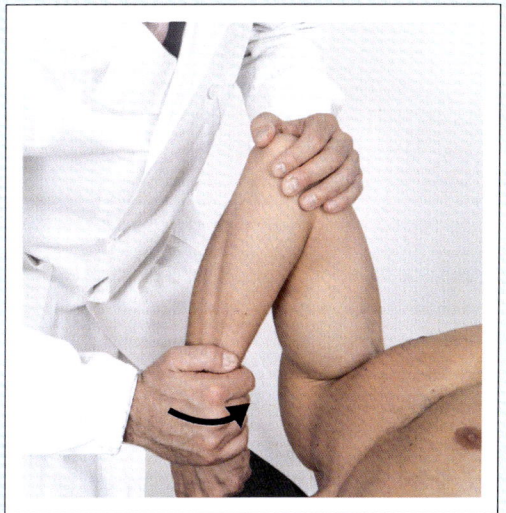

SUPRASPINATUS

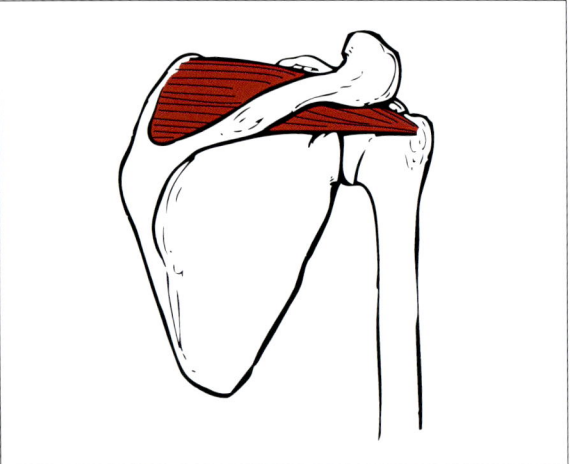

Supraspinatus
Origin: medial two-thirds of supraspinatous fossa of scapula.
Insertion: superior facet on greater tubercle of humerus and capsule of shoulder joint.
Innervation: suprascapular (C5-C6).
Action: abducts humerus (first 15 to 20 degrees); holds head of humerus in glenoid cavity; sometimes acts as an extensor.

Chapman's reflexes
Anterior: over coracoid process
Posterior: base of skull to C1 lamina

Neurovascular point
bregma

Nutrition
brain substance; RNA

Acupuncture meridian association
conception vessel

Common subluxations
C4 and C5

Associated point
T8 and T9 (conception vessel)

Visceral association
brain

CLINICAL*

- pseudo frozen shoulder: limitation in humerus abduction (first 15 to 20 degrees)
- any shoulder pain or shoulder movement problem
- origin and insertion injury in "rotator cuff syndrome"
- brain
- weakness found with CVA including TIA

*Courtesy of Drs. Walter Schmitt and Kerry McCord
Quintessential Applications: A(K) Clinical Protocol (QA)

POSTURE

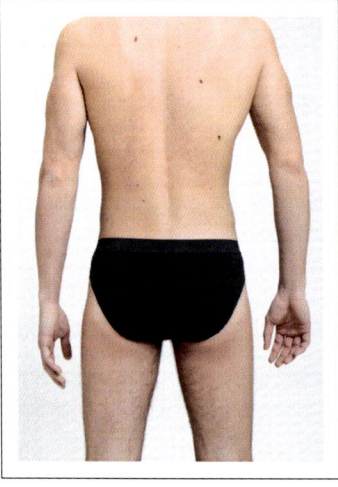

Arm hangs in internal rotation with palm facing posteriorly.

SUPRASPINATUS

Test 1

Position
Supine, seated, or standing.

Test
with teeth lightly clenched and with elbow locked into extension, patient abducts and flexes humerus to approximately 15 degrees to have antecubital fossa facing anteriorly. Examiner stabilizes the superior surface of ipsilateral shoulder with one hand while the other contacts the posterior surface of the distal forearm and uses it as a lever to direct pressure toward adduction and extension of the humerus.

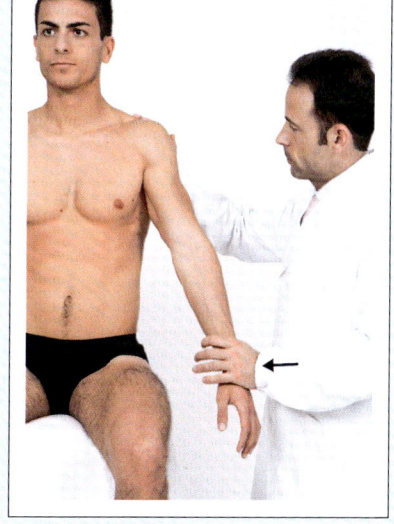

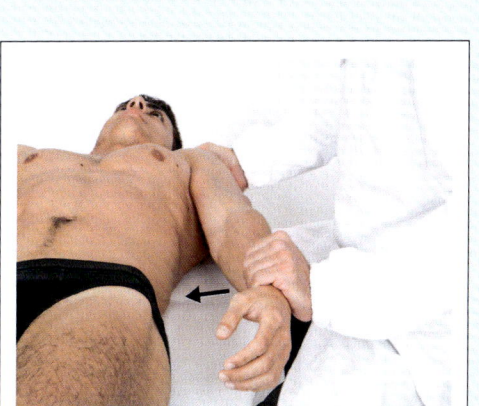

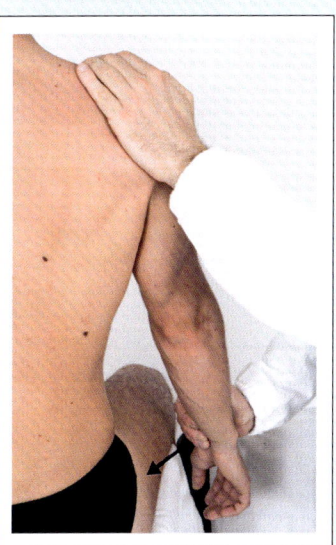

Common error

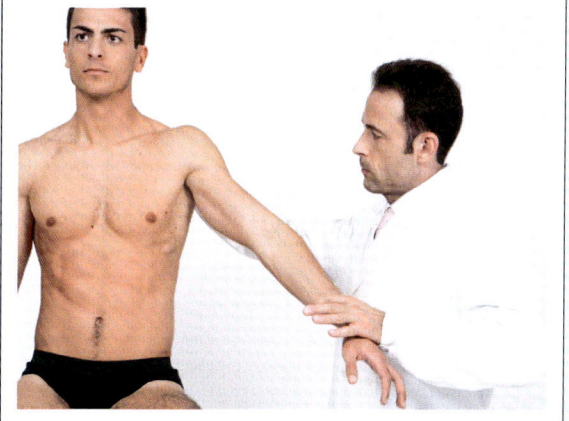

Too much abduction in starting position.

TENSOR FASCIA LATA

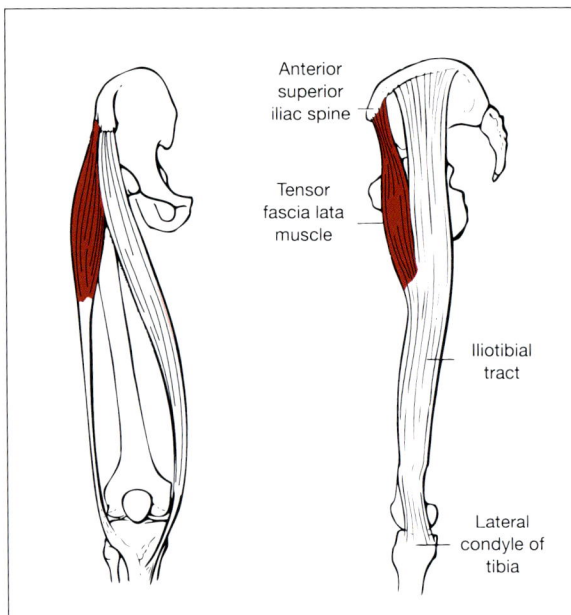

Tensor Fascia Lata
Origin: anterior part of external lip of iliac crest and anterior border of ilium.

Insertion: middle third of the iliotibial tract which inserts into lateral condyle of tibia.

Innervation: superior gluteal (L4-S1).

Action: abducts, internally rotates, and flexes thigh; tenses fascia lata thereby stabilizing the knee laterally.

Chapman's reflexes
Anterior: iliotibial band
Posterior: L2 to L4 to crest of ilium

Neurovascular point
parietal eminence

Nutrition
probiotics; acidophilus; fenugreek, vitamin D; bilateral weakness is associated with iron deficiency

Acupuncture meridian association
large intestine

Common subluxations
L4, L5 and S1

Meric TS line
L4

Associated point
L4 and L5 (large intestine)

Visceral association
large intestine

CLINICAL*

- lateral knee problem
- meralgia paresthetica
- recurrent sacroiliac subluxation
- decreased hip abduction/hip arthritis
- colon problems/dysbiosis

*Courtesy of Drs. Walter Schmitt and Kerry McCord
Quintessential Applications: A(K) Clinical Protocol (QA)

TENSOR FASCIA LATA

POSTURE

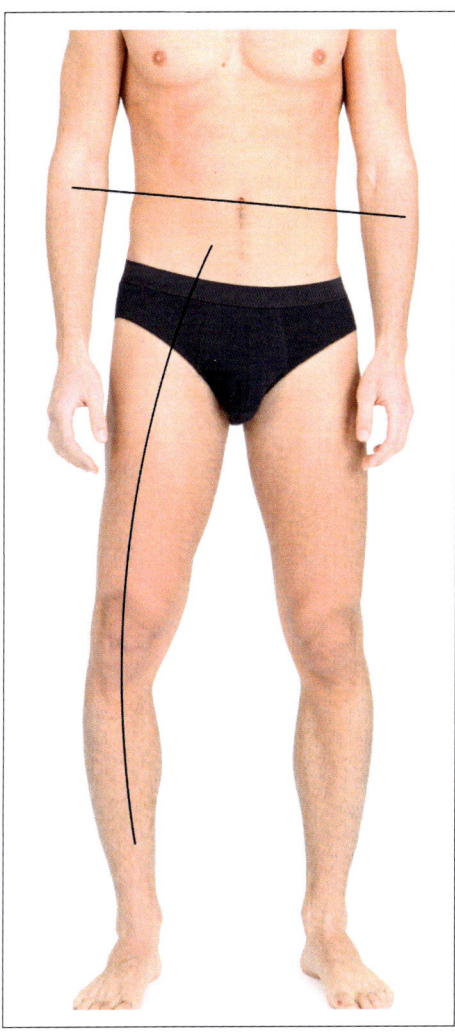

Genu varus and pelvic elevation on weak side.

Test

Position
Supine.

Test
Keeping the knee locked in extension, patient internally rotates, abducts, and flexes femur. Examiner uses one hand to stabilize the opposite leg distally while the other hand contacts the lateral surface of the distal leg on the side being tested and directs pressure toward adduction and extension.

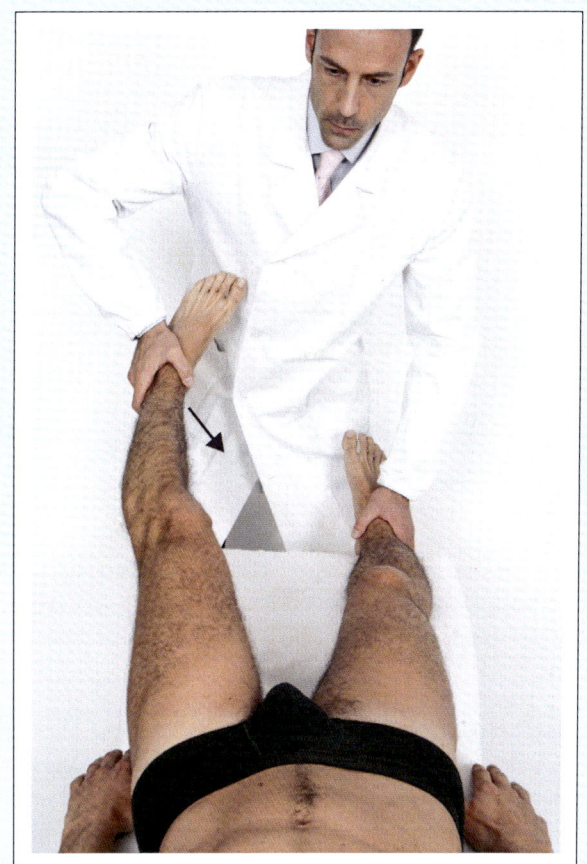

TENSOR FASCIA LATA

Common errors

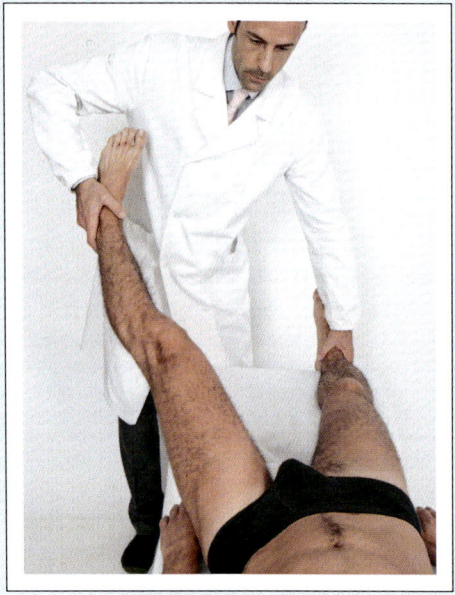
Too much femur abduction.

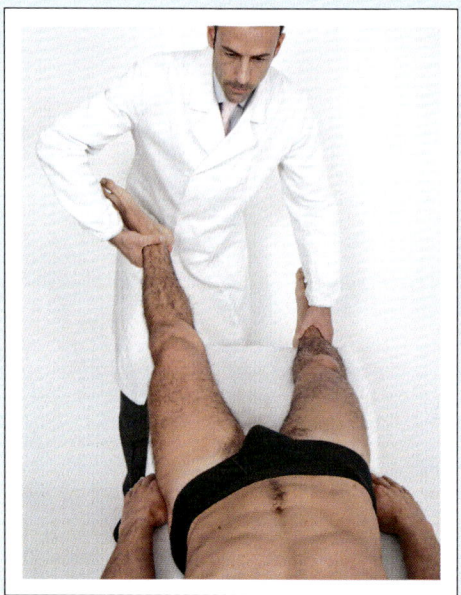
Femur is allowed to laterally rotate.

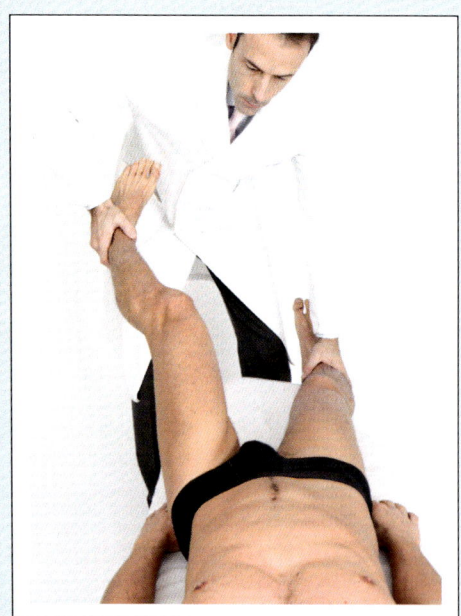
Knee is allowed to bend.

TERES MAJOR

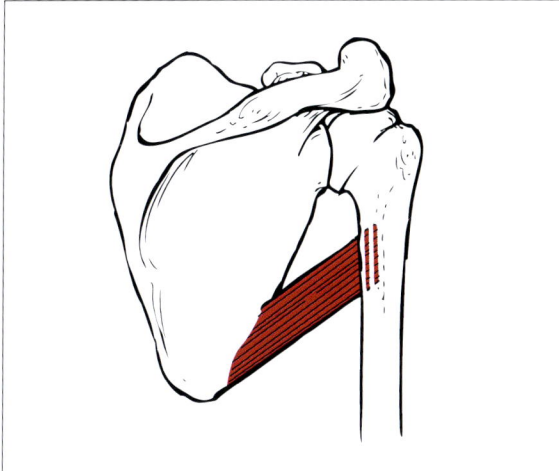

Teres Major
Origin: dorsal surface of inferior angle of scapula and lower one-third of scapular axillary border.
Insertion: medial lip of intertubercular groove of humerus.
Innervation: lower subscapular (C5-C7).
Action: extension of the shoulder joint with internal rotation and some adduction of humerus; stabilizes upper portion of humerus during movement.

CLINICAL[*]

- can raise arm in lateral rotation but not in medial rotation
- difficulty swimming
- associated with drooling and need for Phosphorus and acid-ash minerals
- associated with excessive sweating and need for kelp and other alkaline-ash minerals
- associated with plantar warts related to potassium deficiency
- associated with difficulty tasting related to zinc deficiency
- thoracic fixations when bilaterally weak

[*]Courtesy of Drs. Walter Schmitt and Kerry McCord Quintessential Applications: A(K) Clinical Protocol (QA)

Chapman's reflexes
Anterior: 2nd, 3rd, 4th, and 5th intercostal spaces
Posterior: T2-T3

Neurovascular point 1
1 inch below pterion

Neurovascular point 2
junction of rib 1, clavicle, and sternum

Nutrition
evaluate acid (phosphorus, acid-ash minerals)/alkaline balance (kelp, alkaline ash minerals); acid or alkaline ash minerals; potassium; zinc

Acupuncture meridian association
governing vessel

Common subluxations
C5, C6, and C7; thoracic fixations

Associated point
T7 and T8

Visceral association
generally associated with spine because of its correlation with thoracic vertebrae fixations

TERES MAJOR

POSTURE

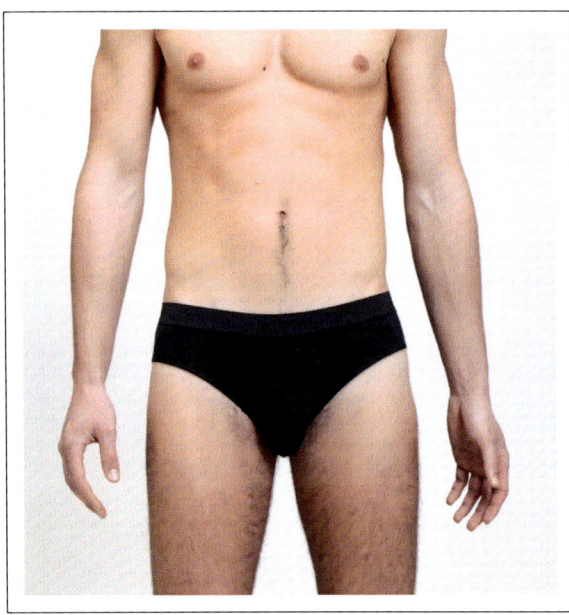

Arm, forearm, and hand hang in lateral rotation, palm rotated toward the front.

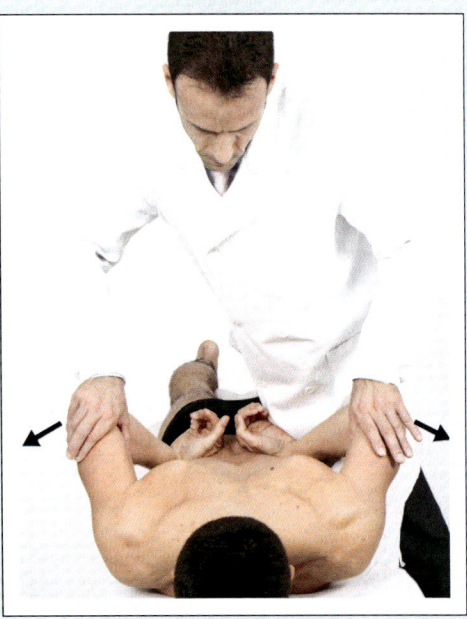

Test

Position
Prone.

Test
With the forearm flexed to about 90 degrees, patient slightly abducts (20 to 30 degrees), extends (20 to 30 degrees), then internally rotates humerus to have dorsal surface of the hand resting over the ipsilateral posterior iliac crest.
Examiner contacts the medial surface of the distal humerus and directs pressure toward abduction and flexion of the humerus.

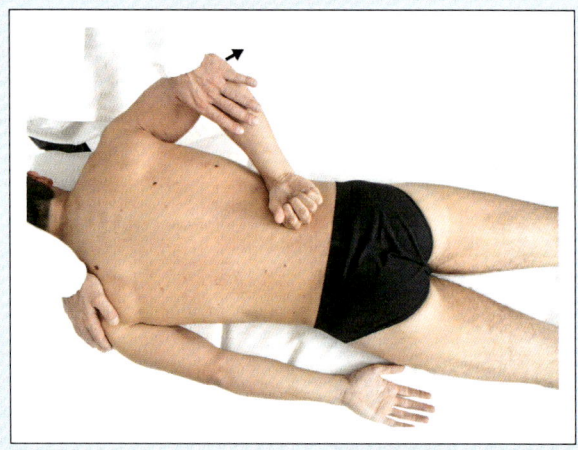

N.B.
The test is often performed bilaterally.

TERES MAJOR

Common errors

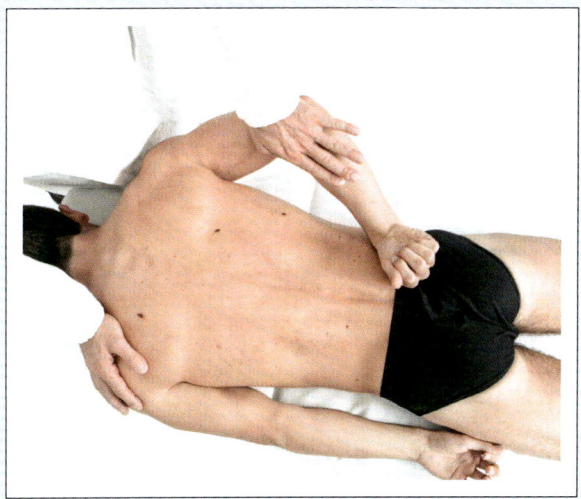

Patient's hand therapy localizes sacroilliac joint or lumbar vertebrae.

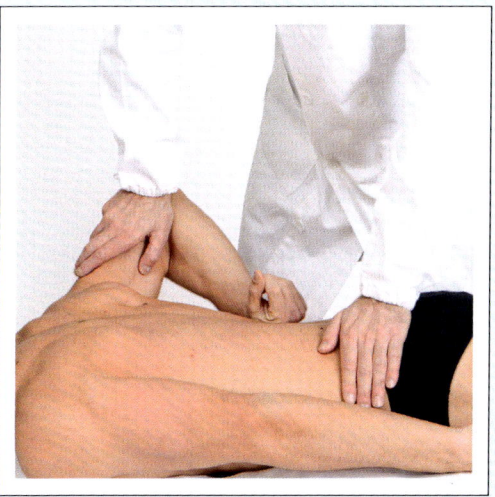

Too much extension of humerus.

TERES MINOR

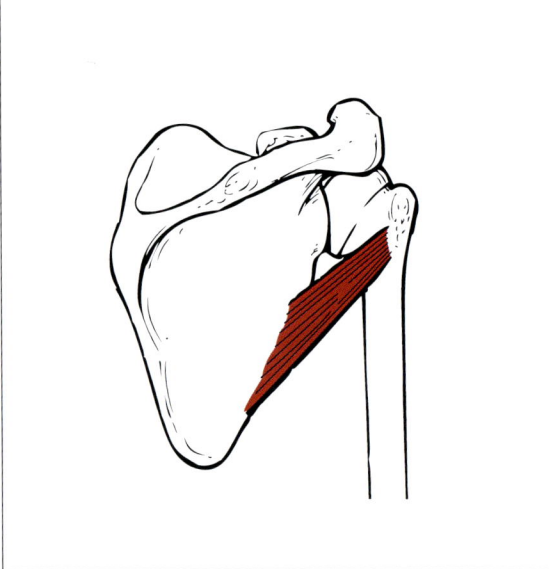

Teres Minor
Origin: superior two-thirds of dorsal surface of the lateral border of scapula.

Insertion: inferior facet on greater tubercle of humerus.

Innervation: axillary (C4-C6).

Action: external rotation of humerus; slight adduction and extension of humerus; stabilizes head of humerus in glenoid cavity during movement; assists deltoid in humerus abduction.

CLINICAL*

- difficulty elevating shoulder
- difficulty reaching backward
- can't raise arm over head with palm up
- difficulty playing tennis (backhand), golf, etc.
- origin and insertion injury in "rotator cuff syndrome"
- thyroid

*Courtesy of Drs. Walter Schmitt and Kerry McCord Quintessential Applications: A(K) Clinical Protocol (QA)

Chapman's reflexes
Anterior: 2nd intercostal space
Posterior: T2 and T3

Neurovascular point
1 inch below the pterion and at the junction of the clavicle, sternum, and rib 1

Nutrition
iodine; thyroid tissue; parotid tissue

Acupuncture meridian association
triple heater

Common subluxations
C5 and C6

Associated point
L1 and L2 triple warmer

Visceral association
thyroid

TERES MINOR

POSTURE

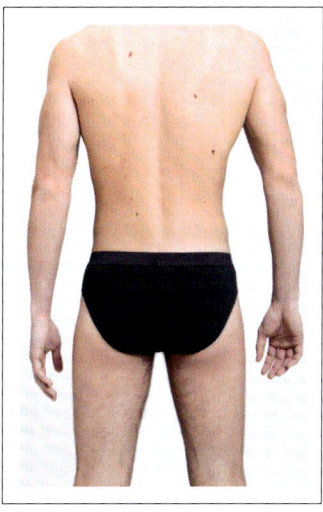

Arm, forearm, and hand hang in internal rotation with palm facing backward.

Test

Position
Seated or supine.

Test
Patient lightly clenches teeth, flexes forearm to 90 degrees, and externally rotates humerus. Examiner stabilizes the elbow with one hand, while the other hand contacts the posterior, distal forearm and uses it as a lever to direct pressure toward internal rotation of the humerus.

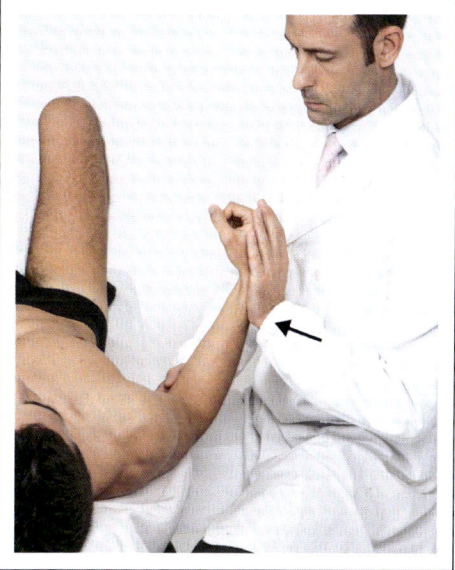

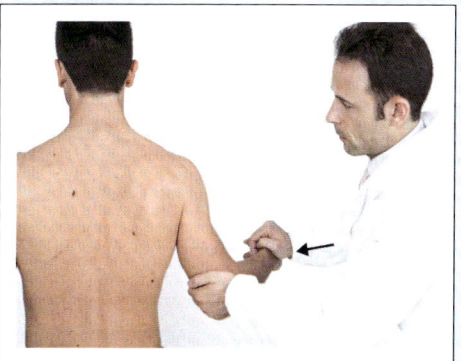

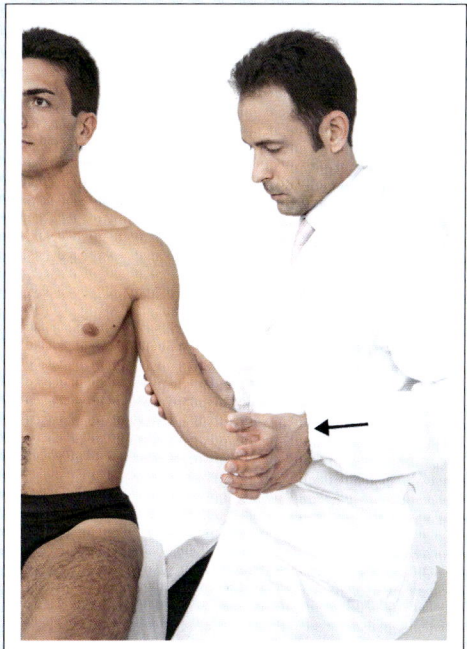

TIBIALIS ANTERIOR

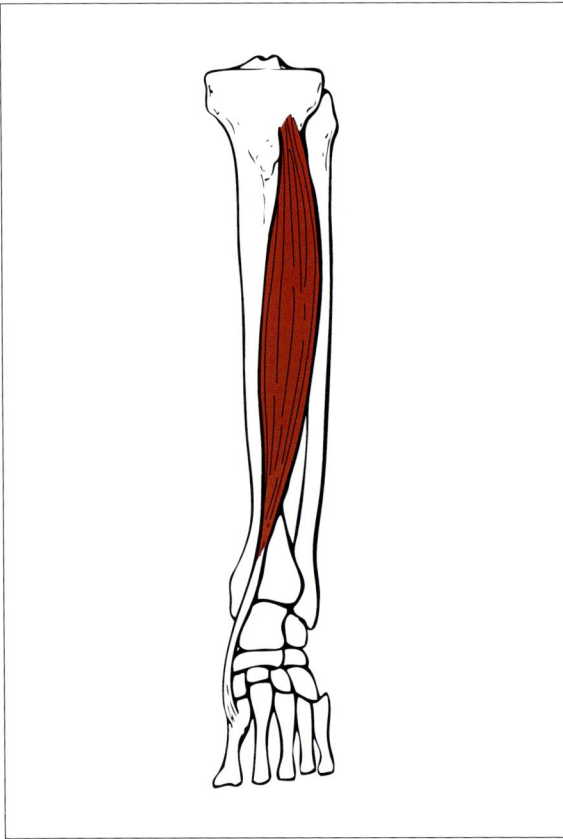

Tibialis Anterior
Origin: lateral condyle and superior half of lateral surface of tibia.

Insertion: medial and plantar surfaces of medial cuneiform; base of first metatarsal.

Innervation: peroneal (L4-S1).

Action: dorsiflexes and inverts foot.

Chapman's reflexes
Anterior: superior pubic bone
Posterior: L2

Neurovascular point
bilateral frontal bone eminences

Nutrition
vitamins A, C, and P combinations (bladder infections); vitamin B ("B" and "G")

Acupuncture meridian association
bladder

Common subluxations
L4, L5, and S1

Associated point
sacrum (S1), (bladder)

Visceral association
urinary bladder

CLINICAL*

- foot drop
- catching toes in carpet
- stubbing toes
- high stepping gait
- anterior shin splints
- bladder

*Courtesy of Drs. Walter Schmitt and Kerry McCord
Quintessential Applications: A(K) Clinical Protocol (QA)

TIBIALIS ANTERIOR

Test

Position
Supine or seated.

Test
With teeth lightly clenched, and toes in flexion, patient inverts and dorsiflexes foot. Examiner uses one hand to stabilize just proximal to the lateral malleolus, while the other hand contacts the medial, dorsal surface of the foot to direct pressure toward plantarflexion and eversion.

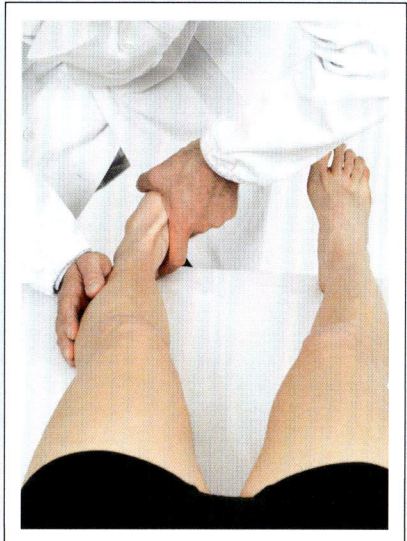
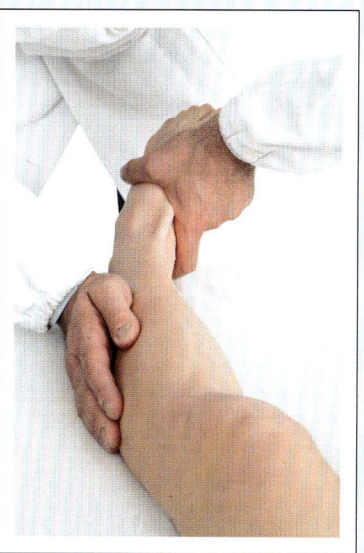

POSTURE

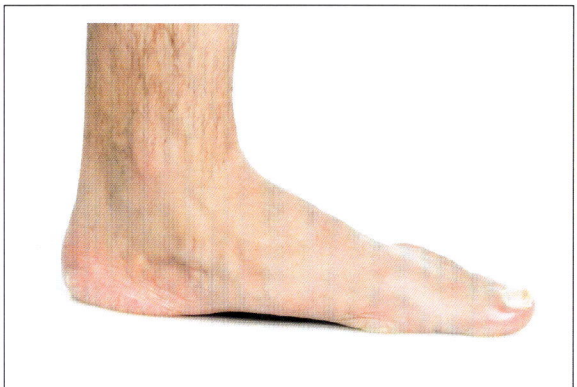

Pes planus "flat feet" and/or foot pronation.

Common error

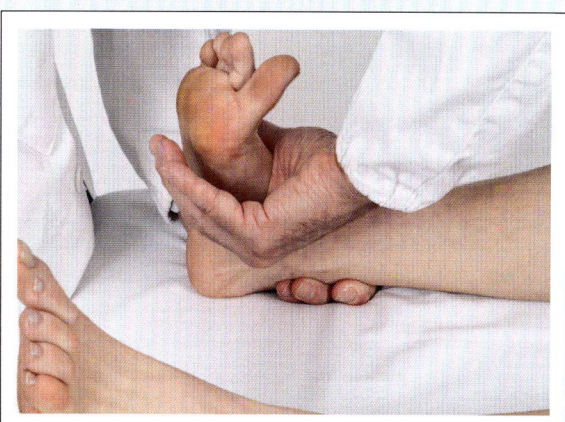

Toes are allowed to extend.

TRAPEZIUS LOWER DIVISION

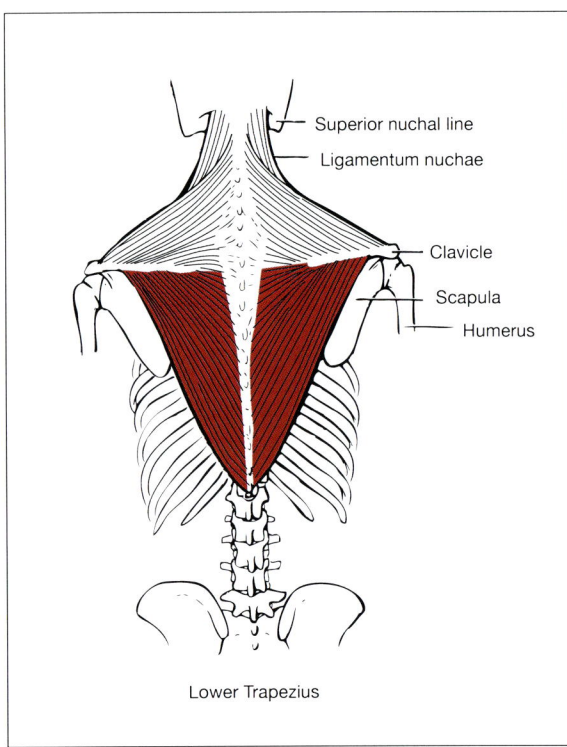

Lower Trapezius

Trapezius Lower Division
Origin: spinous processes of T6-T12.

Insertion: medial third of the spine of scapula.

Innervation: spinal accessory (CN XI); ventral rami of C2-C4.

Action: depresses scapula and gives it inferior stabilization; draws acromion posteriorly; assists in maintaining spine in extension; acting with the upper trapezius creates superior rotation of scapula.

Chapman's reflexes
Anterior: left 7th and 8th intercostal spaces
Posterior: left T7 and T8

Neurovascular point
1 inch superior to lambda

Nutrition
spleen substance; vitamin C; calcium

Acupuncture meridian association
spleen/pancreas

Common subluxations
C2, C3, and C4

Meric TS line
T7

Associated point
T11, T12

Visceral association
spleen

CLINICAL*

- difficulty raising arm over head
- when unilaterally weak, lower thoracic scoliosis
- when bilaterally weak, increased thoracic kyphosis
- when bilaterally weak, lumbo-thoracic vertebral fixations
- difficulty standing at attention
- opposite shoulder problem due to tight contralateral trapezius

*Courtesy of Drs. Walter Schmitt and Kerry McCord
Quintessential Applications: A(K) Clinical Protocol (QA)

TRAPEZIUS LOWER DIVISION

POSTURE

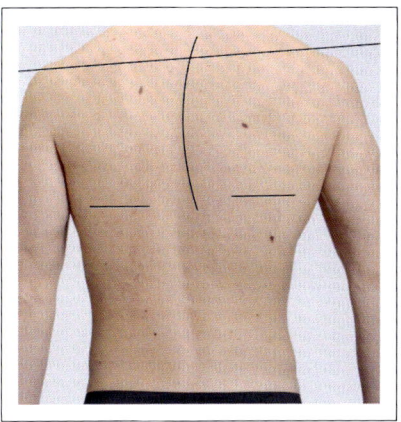

Unilateral weakness: ipsilateral shoulder and scapula elevated with shoulder rollled forward; thoracic scoliosis (concave on weak side).

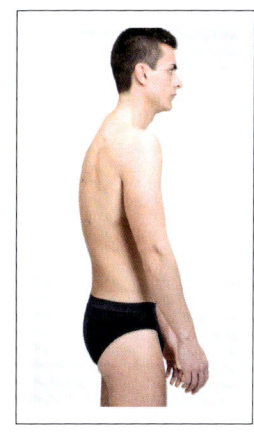

Bilateral weakness: increased thoracic kyphosis with both shoulders rolled forward.

Test 1

Position
Prone.

Test
With elbow locked in extension, the prone patient abducts (140 degrees) and externally rotates humerus so that the thumb points upward toward the ceiling. Examiner stabilizes with one hand over the contralateral, posterior iliac crest, while the other hand contacts the lateral surface of the distal humerus or distal forearm, and directs pressure straight down toward the floor. In this way the arm is used as a lever to impart pressure toward abduction of the scapula.

N.B.
To determine if this muscle tests weak, examiner must observe for abduction of the scapula away from the spine, as opposed to evaluating whether humerus can resist test pressure.

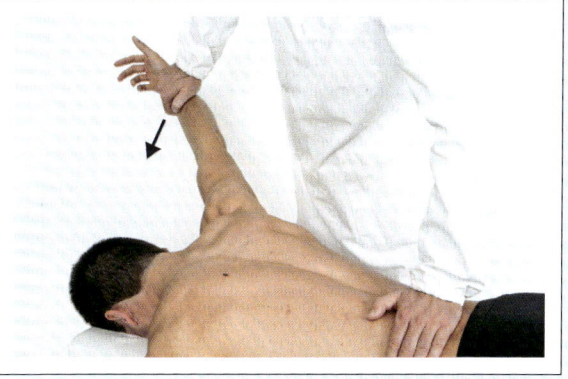

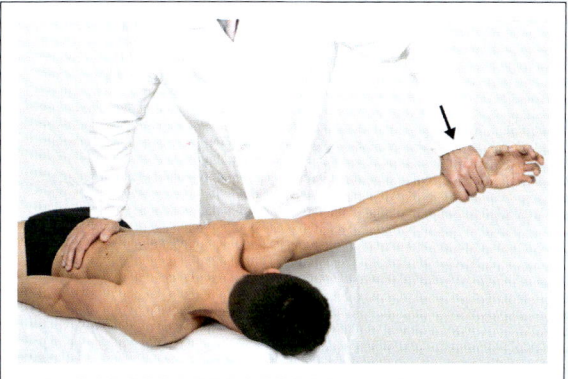

TRAPEZIUS LOWER DIVISION

Test 2

Position
Prone.

Test
With elbow locked in extension, supine patient abducts (140 degrees), and externally rotates the humerus so that the thumb points downward toward the floor. Examiner contacts the lateral surface of the distal forearm and directs pressure straight upward toward the ceiling. In this way the arm is used as a lever to impart pressure toward abduction of the scapula.

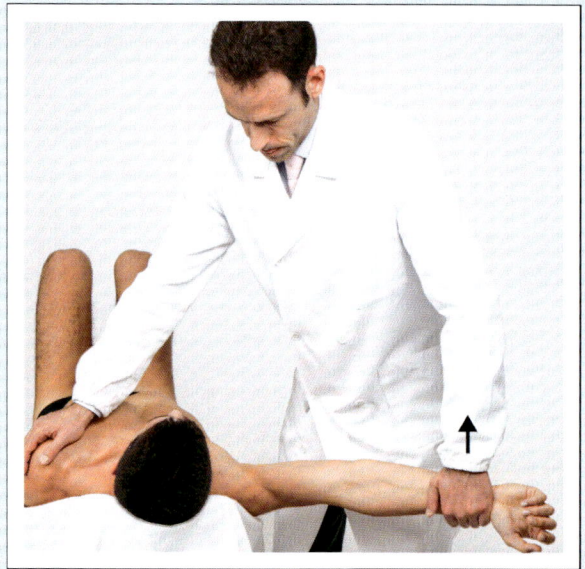

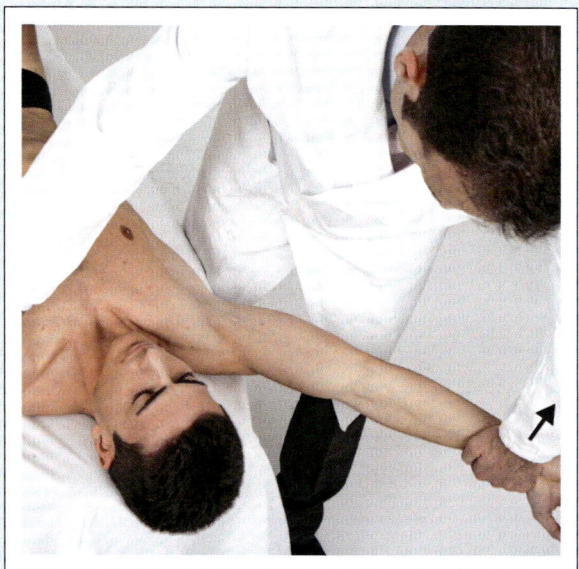

TRAPEZIUS MIDDLE DIVISION

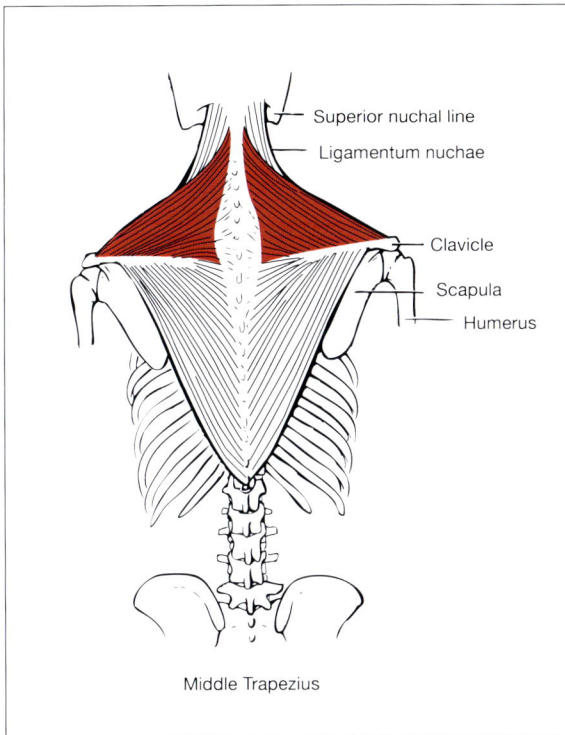

Middle Trapezius

Trapezius Middle Division

Origin: spinous processes of T1-T5.

Insertion: superior border of spine of scapula.

Innervation: spinal accessory (CN XI); ventral rami of (C2-C4).

Action: adducts, retracts, and slightly elevates scapula bringing it medially toward the spine; draws acromion process posteriorly; braces shoulder girdle.

Chapman's reflexes
Anterior: left 7th and 8th intercostal space
Posterior: left T7 and T8

Neurovascular point
1 inch superior to lambda

Nutrition
vitamin C; spleen substance; calcium

Acupuncture meridian association
spleen/pancreas

Common subluxations
C2, C3, and C4

Meric TS line
T7

Associated point
T11, T12

Visceral association
spleen

CLINICAL*

- difficulty standing at attention
- opposite shoulder problem due to tight contralateral middle trapezius

*Courtesy of Drs. Walter Schmitt and Kerry McCord
Quintessential Applications: A(K) Clinical Protocol (QA)

TRAPEZIUS MIDDLE DIVISION

POSTURE

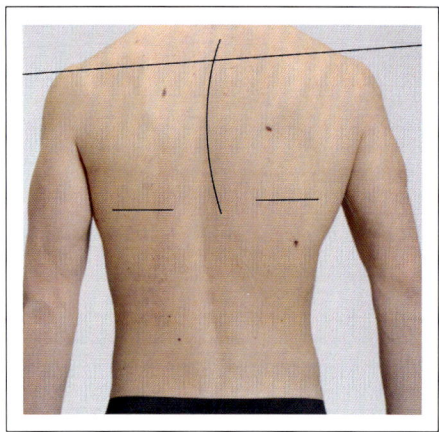

Unilateral weakness: thoracic spine scoliosis concave on the side of weakness.

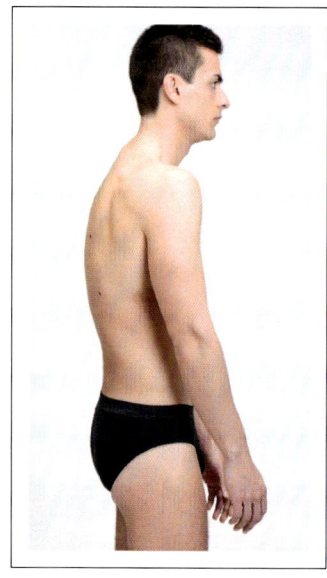

Bilateral weakness: increased thoracic kyphosis.

Test 1

Position Prone.

Test
Prone patient locks elbow into extension, abducts shoulder to 90 degrees, and externally rotates humerus so that thumb points upward toward the ceiling. Examiner stabilizes with one hand over the contralateral scapula, while the other hand contacts the lateral surface of the distal humerus or distal forearm, and directs pressure straight down toward the floor. In this way the humerus is used as a lever to impart pressure toward abduction of the scapula.

N.B. To determine if this muscle tests weak, examiner must observe for abduction of the scapula away from the spine, as opposed to evaluating whether humerus can resist test pressure.

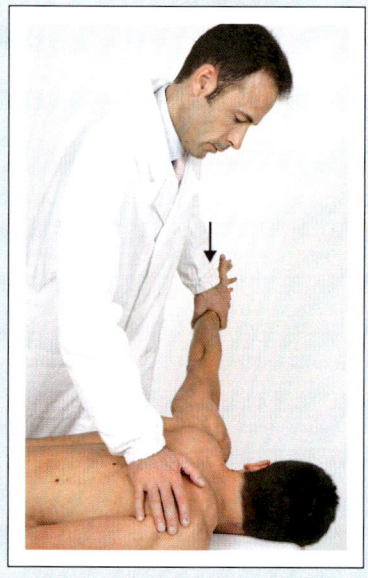

TRAPEZIUS MIDDLE DIVISION

Test 2

Position
Supine.

Test
Supine patient locks elbow into extension, abducts shoulder to 90 degrees, and externally rotates humerus so that thumb points down toward the floor. Examiner contacts the lateral surface of the distal forearm and uses it as a lever pulling straight upward toward the ceiling to impart pressure toward abduction of the scapula.

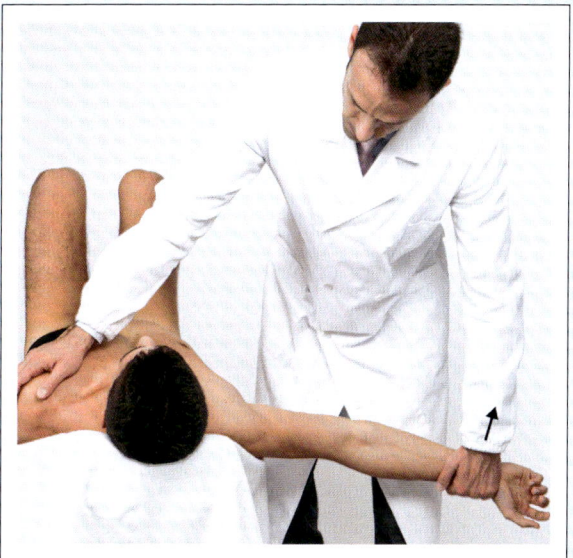

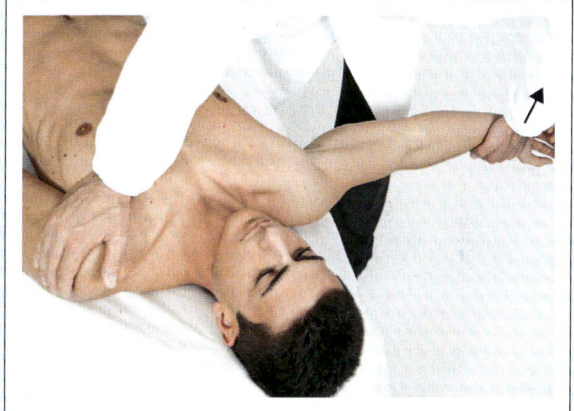

TRAPEZIUS UPPER DIVISION

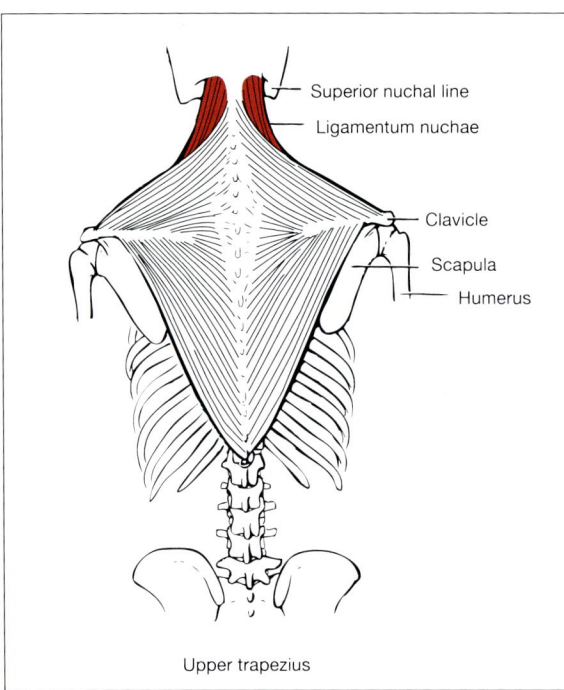

Upper trapezius

Trapezius Upper Division
Origin: external occipital protuberance; medial third of superior nuchal line; ligamentum nuchae; spinous process of C7 vertebra.

Insertion: lateral third of clavicle; acromion; spine of scapula.

Innervation: spinal accessory (CN XI); ventral ramus of C2-C4.

Action: rotates scapula so glenoid cavity faces superiorly; adducts scapula when acting with other divisions of trapezius; rotates head to opposite side.

CLINICAL*

- difficulty turning neck to opposite side as with looking over shoulder to back up car
- difficulty (pain and decreased range of motion) with lateral neck flexion as with holding ear to phone
- upper trapezius pain either due to contralateral upper trapezius inhibition or ipsilateral to latissimus dorsi inhibition
- pain in ipsilateral or contralateral levator scapula
- difficulty with shoulder (glenoid fossa) elevation
- eye and ear

*Courtesy of Drs. Walter Schmitt and Kerry McCord Quintessential Applications: A(K) Clinical Protocol (QA)

Chapman's reflexes
Anterior: 1 inch band - 3 inches long over the anterior, upper arm
Posterior: nuchal line/C1

Neurovascular point
over zygomatic process at the temporosphenoidal junction

Nutrition
vitamins A, B, F, and G; calcium

Acupuncture meridian association
kidney

Common subluxations
cervical, cranial faults

Associated point
L2, L3 (kidney)

Visceral association
eye and ear

TRAPEZIUS UPPER DIVISION

POSTURE

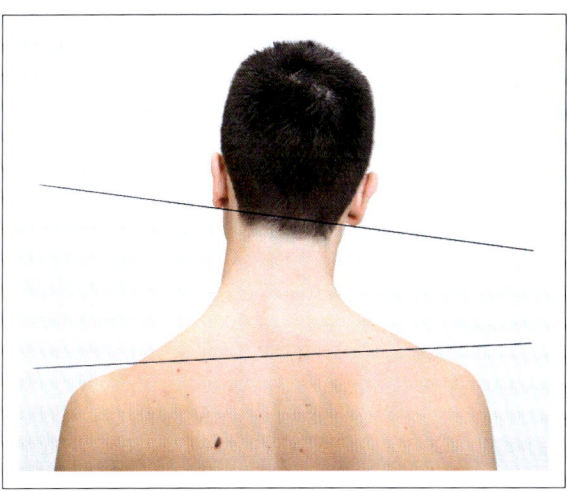

Occiput and shoulder separated (ear high and shoulder low on weak side).

Test 1

Position
Best tested seated but can also be performed supine or standing.

Test
Seated patient lightly clenches teeth, then elevates shoulder, bringing it toward the ear, while simultaneously laterally flexing neck to bring the ear toward the shoulder. The head is then rotated toward the opposite shoulder to approximately 20 degrees.

Examiner places one hand on the superior surface of the shoulder and the other on the postero-lateral head. Force is then directed through both hands in the direction of reducing the approximation of the head and shoulder.

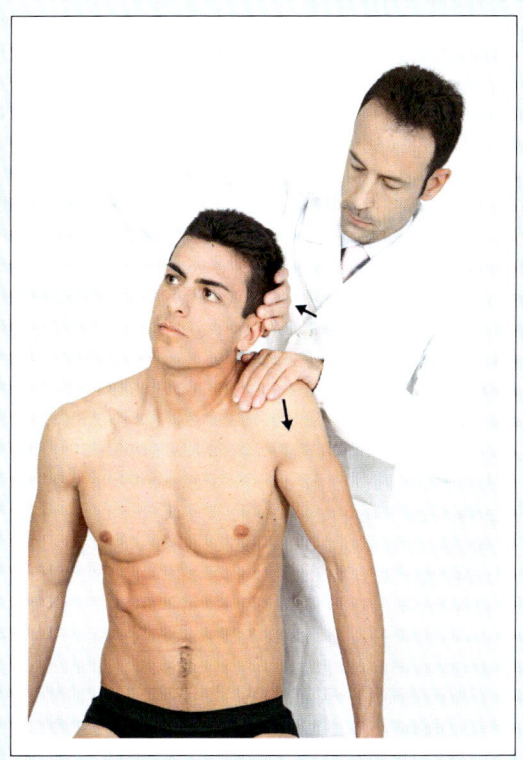
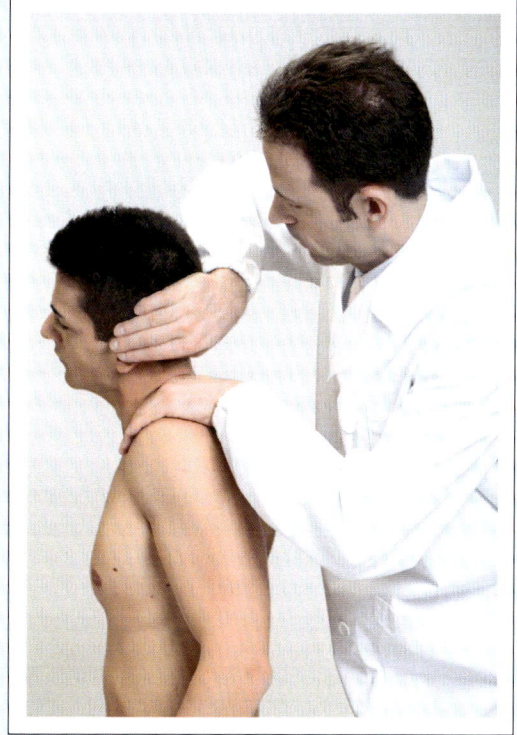

TRAPEZIUS UPPER DIVISION

Common errors

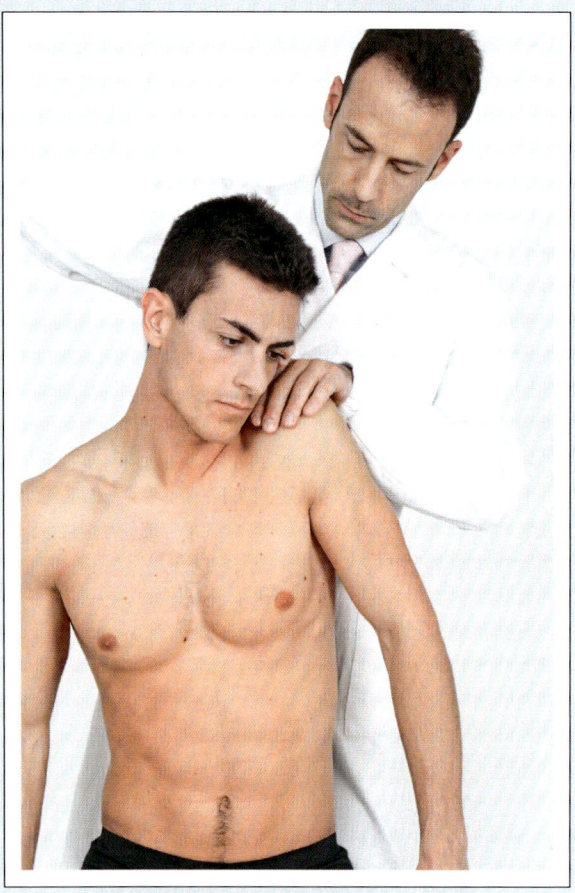

Head is allowed to rotate toward side being tested.

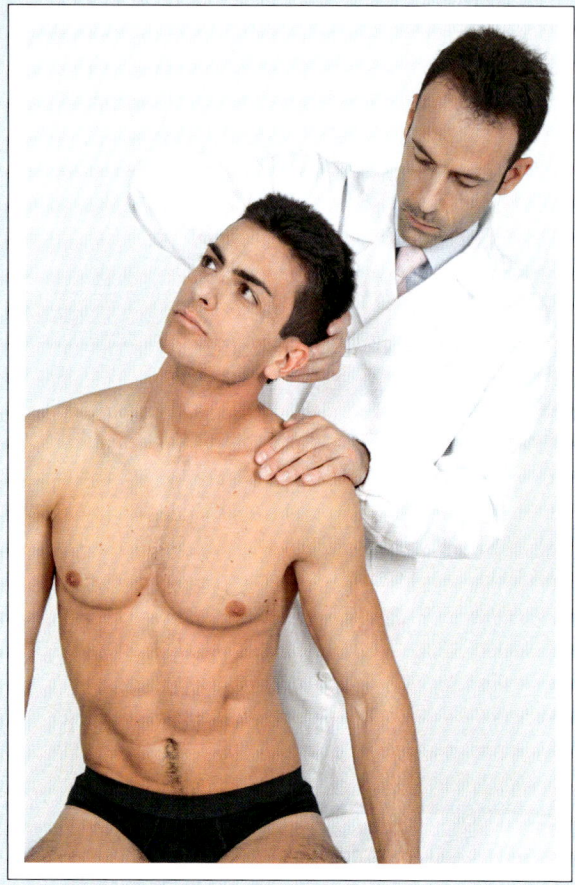

Shoulder is not elevated.

TRICEPS BRACHII

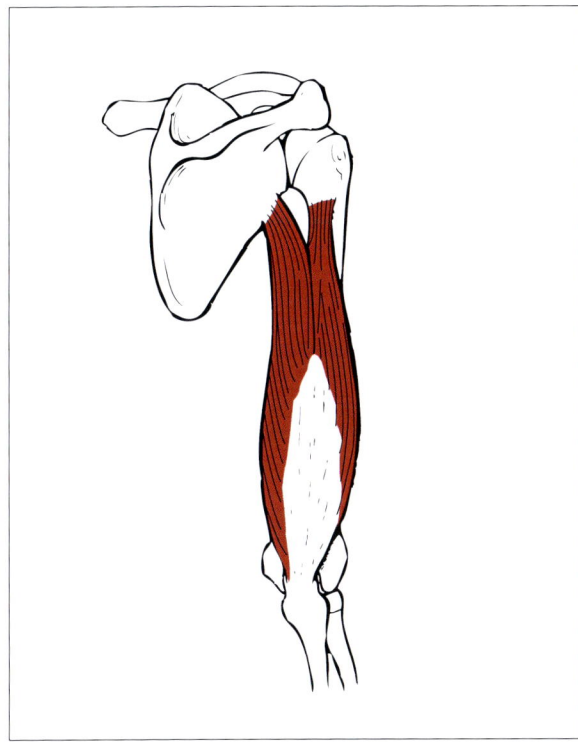

Triceps Brachii
Origin long head: infraglenoid tubercle of scapula.

Origin lateral head: postero-lateral surface of humerus.

Origin medial head: lower posterior surface of humerus.

Insertion: olecranon process of ulna.

Innervation: radial (C6-C8).

Action: extends forearm;
long head of triceps steadies superior portion of abducted humerus and aids in adducting and extending the arm.

Chapman's reflexes
Anterior: left 7th intercostal space
Posterior: left T-7/8

Neurovascular point
squamous suture directly over the ear

Nutrition
betaine hydrochloride;
pancreas concentrate of nucleoprotein extract, zinc, glucose regulation related substances (chromium, vanadium, etc.), vitamin A and vitamin F

Acupuncture meridian association
spleen

Common subluxations
C6-T1

Meric TS line
T6

Associated point
T11, T12 (spleen/pancreas)

Visceral association
pancreas

TRICEPS BRACHII

CLINICAL*
Medial and Lateral Heads

- elbow problems (tennis and golf elbow)
- difficulty (pain and decreased range of motion) with resisted shoulder extension
- weak with cervical radiculopathies
- overfacillated in hyperinsulism

*Courtesy of Drs. Walter Schmitt and Kerry McCord
Quintessential Applications: A(K) Clinical Protocol (QA)

CLINICAL*
Long Head

- elbow problems
- difficulty (pain and decreased range of motion) of shoulder
- difficulty with the motion of elbowing someone behind you
- overfacillated in hyperinsulism

*Courtesy of Drs. Walter Schmitt and Kerry McCord
Quintessential Applications: A(K) Clinical Protocol (QA)

POSTURE

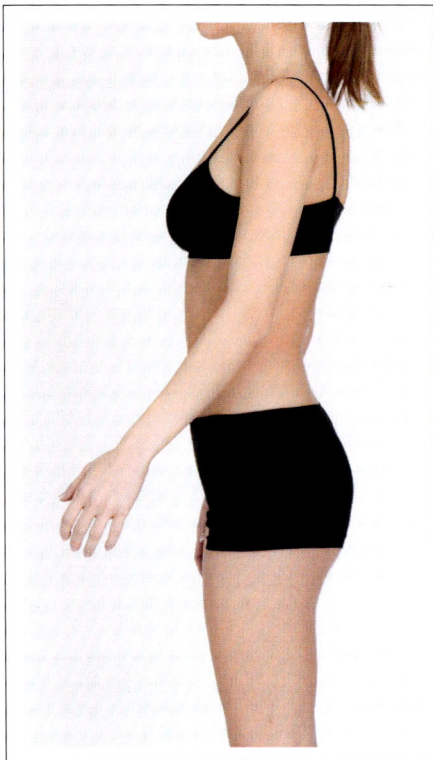

Arm and forearm hang in slight flexion.

TRICEPS BRACHII

Test

Position Seated or supine.

Test
Patient lightly clenches teeth, fully supinates forearm, flexes it to about 45 degrees, then abducts (30 to 40 degrees) and slightly externally rotates humerus. Examiner uses one hand to stabilize at the elbow while the other hand contacts the posterior, distal forearm, and directs pressure toward forearm flexion.

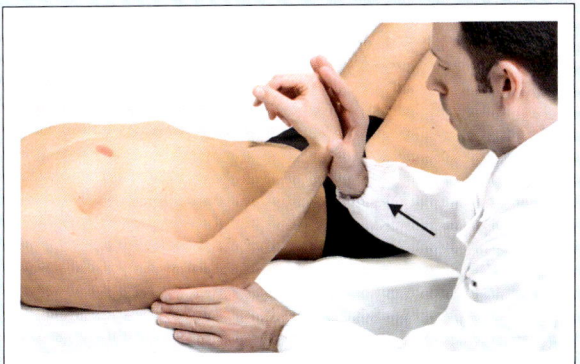

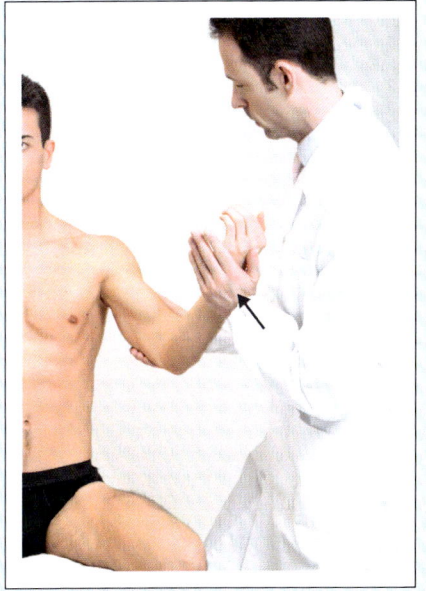

Common errors

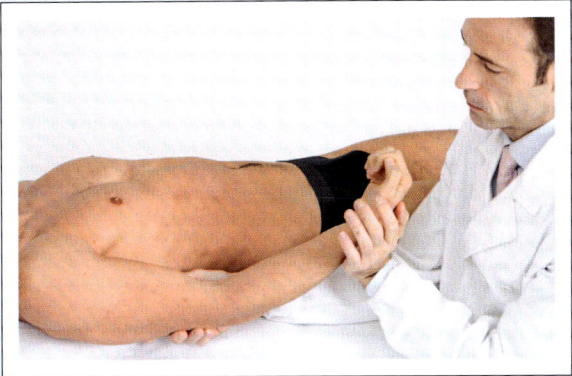

Excess humerus extension.

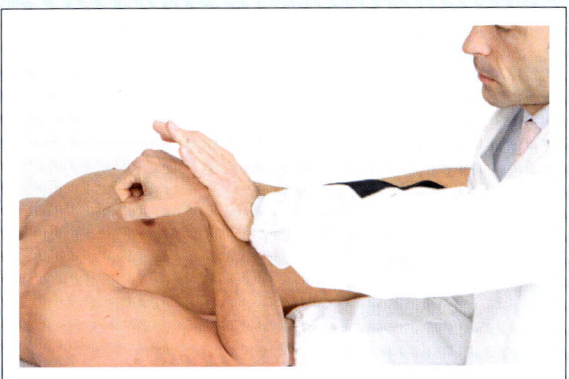

Excess humerus flexion.

TRICEPS BRACHII

Test for Long head of Triceps Brachii

Position
Seated or supine.

Test
Patient fully supinates forearm and flexes it to 90 degrees. Examiner contacts posterior, distal humerus and directs pressure toward flexion.

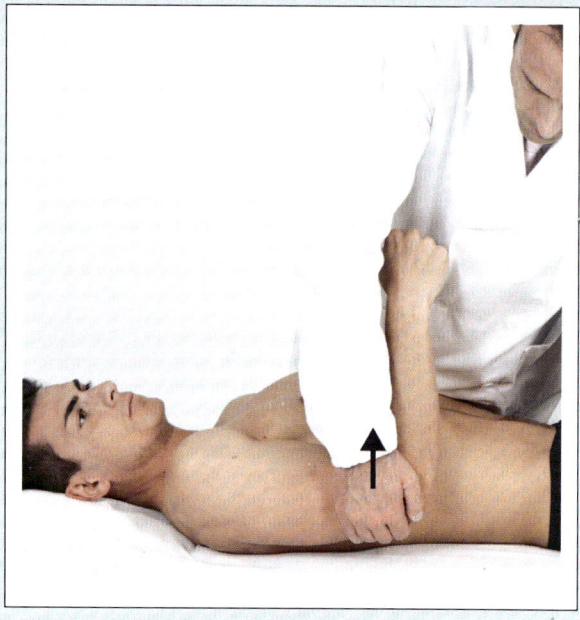

Common error

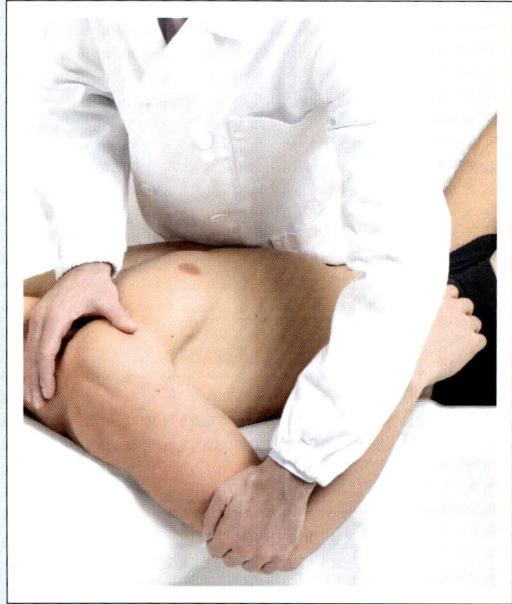

Excess humerus extension.